Black Seed Oil Guide

Harnessing Nature's Secret
for Optimal Wellness

Unlock the Power of Black Seed Oil
for Health, Beauty, and Culinary Delights

Jasmine Bloomfield

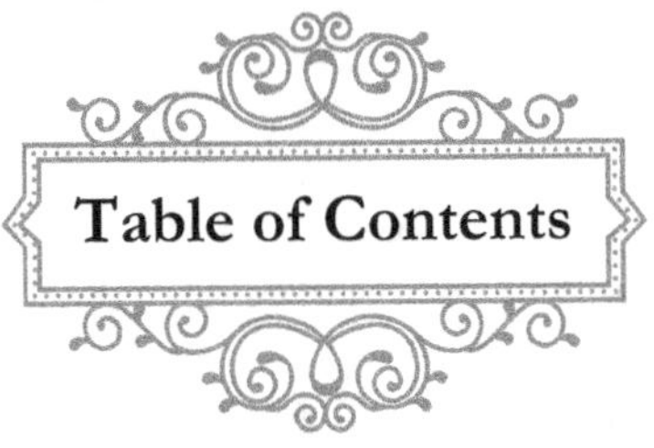

Table of Contents

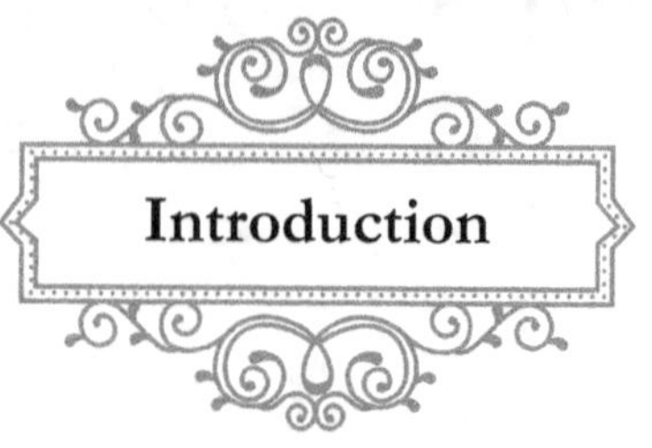

Introduction

Purpose of the Book

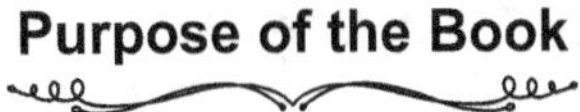

The purpose of this book is to provide a comprehensive guide to black seed oil, offering valuable knowledge to help you navigate the complexities of this remarkable natural remedy.

Our aim is to share the numerous benefits of black seed oil and empower you to incorporate it seamlessly into your daily routine. Whether you are dealing with inflammation, striving to improve the health of your skin and hair, or simply seeking a greater sense of vitality, this book will be your trusted companion on the journey to optimal well-being.

By demystifying the science behind black seed oil and providing clear, actionable guidance, we aim to equip you with the knowledge and confidence to harness its transformative power.

So, dear reader, I invite you to embark on this enlightening journey with an open mind and a sense of curiosity. Let us together explore and discover the wisdom of black seed oil, guided by the shared commitment to vibrant health and vitality. However, our purpose goes beyond just providing instruction.

We also seek to foster a sense of community, to encourage the embrace of nature's healing gifts and to regain control over our health destinies. As you delve into the pages of this guide, you will not only deepen your understanding of black seed oil, but also become part of a global community of like-minded individuals dedicated to holistic living.

Within these pages, you will find a wealth of insights, tips, and practical advice that have been gathered from years of dedicated study and personal experience. Our goal is not only to inform, but also to inspire and instill in you a deep appreciation for the incredible potential of black seed oil.

Overview of Black Seed Oil and its Benefits

Get ready to embark on a captivating journey into the world of black seed oil, which holds a wealth of wellness just waiting to be explored. Black seed oil, derived from the seeds of the Nigella sativa plant, has a long history rooted in ancient healing traditions. It has been revered across cultures and civilizations for centuries, and its natural healing properties continue to amaze us today. So, dear reader, I invite you to join me on this voyage of discovery into the essence of black seed oil and the limitless potential it holds. Together, let us unlock the secrets of this extraordinary elixir and embrace a future filled with health, vitality, and holistic well-being. Black seed oil is packed with bioactive compounds like thymoquinone, nigellone, and antioxidants, all of which contribute to its ability to support health and vitality. It offers a wide range of benefits, from its well-known anti-inflammatory properties to its ability to boost the immune system. The advantages of black seed oil are not only diverse but also profound. But the journey doesn't stop there. As you delve deeper into the intricacies of black seed oil, you will uncover its versatility as a skincare product, a hair treatment, and a delicious addition to your culinary creations. From soothing irritated skin to adding a depth of flavor to your favorite dishes, the possibilities are endless and limited only by your imagination. In this guide, you will discover the many ways in which black seed oil can enhance your life. Whether you're looking for relief from common ailments or striving to improve your overall well-being, black seed oil provides a holistic solution that draws on the wisdom of nature.

How to Use This Guide

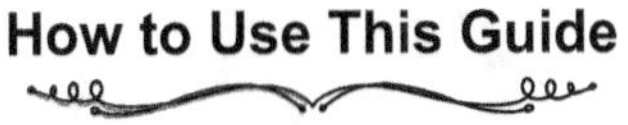

This is your guide to confidently navigate the world of black seed oil. As you begin this enlightening journey, I will provide guidance on how to effectively use the wealth of information in this book. Approach this guide with an open mind and a curious spirit.

Embrace the opportunity to expand your knowledge and understanding of black seed oil and its many benefits.

Familiarize yourself with the structure of the book, as each chapter offers comprehensive insights into different aspects of black seed oil.

Actively engage with the material by taking notes, highlighting key points, and reflecting on how you can apply the wisdom in your own life.

Use the provided references and resources to explore further beyond the text.

Remember that this guide is not just an informational source, but a catalyst for action. Consider how you can use the knowledge gained to improve your health and overall well-being.

With these principles in mind, I invite you to embark on this journey with enthusiasm and curiosity.

Let us discover the secrets of black seed oil together and embrace a future filled with natural wellness and vitality.

Understanding Black Seed Oil

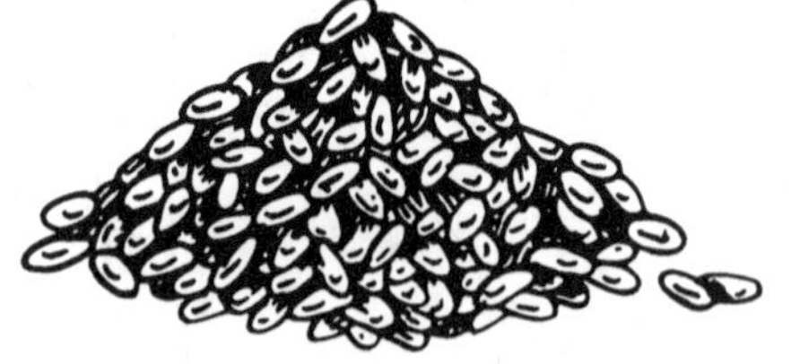

Introduction to Black Seed Oil

Welcome to the fascinating world of black seed oil, an ancient remedy with modern-day relevance that continues to captivate enthusiasts of natural wellness worldwide.

Black seed oil, also known as Nigella sativa oil or black cumin seed oil, is extracted from the seeds of the Nigella sativa plant, native to Southwest Asia. This plant has been revered for its medicinal properties for thousands of years, with references to its use dating back to ancient Egypt and beyond.

At the heart of black seed oil's potency lies its rich composition of bioactive compounds, including thymoquinone, nigellone, and antioxidants. These compounds work synergistically to confer a wide range of health benefits, from anti-inflammatory and immune-boosting effects to potential protective effects against certain diseases.

Key Points to Explore Further:

- Historical significance and cultural use of black seed oil
- Composition and nutritional profile of black seed oil
- Extraction methods and quality considerations
- Health benefits supported by scientific evidence
- Applications in skincare, haircare, and culinary arts

As we delve deeper into the following chapters, we will unravel the mysteries surrounding black seed oil, exploring its diverse applications and uncovering the science behind its remarkable effects on health and well-being. Join me on this journey of discovery as we unlock the potential of black seed oil together.

Historical Background and Cultural Significance

Ancient Origins:

The history of black seed oil traces back to ancient civilizations, where it was revered for its remarkable healing properties. References to black seed oil can be found in ancient Egyptian texts, including the famous Ebers Papyrus, which dates back to around 1550 BCE. In these texts, black seed oil was hailed as a remedy for various ailments, from digestive issues to respiratory complaints.

Medieval Era:

During the medieval period, black seed oil continued to play a prominent role in traditional medicine across the Middle East and beyond. Islamic scholars and physicians such as Avicenna and Ibn Qayyim al-Jawziyya extolled its virtues, citing its efficacy in treating a wide range of conditions.

Renaissance and Beyond:

With the dawn of the Renaissance, interest in herbal medicine experienced a resurgence in Europe, leading to increased exploration of black seed oil's therapeutic potential. European travelers to the Middle East encountered black seed oil and brought back tales of its healing powers, further fueling its popularity.

Modern Revival:

In recent decades, scientific research has shed light on the bioactive compounds found in black seed oil and their potential health benefits. This has led to a modern revival of interest in black seed oil as a natural remedy for various ailments, from inflammation and allergies to skin conditions and beyond.

Cultural Significance:

The cultural significance of black seed oil extends far beyond its medicinal properties. In many cultures, black seed oil is revered as a symbol of health, prosperity, and protection. It is often used in religious ceremonies and rituals, with references to its benefits found in ancient religious texts.

Today, black seed oil continues to be valued for its holistic approach to wellness, drawing upon centuries of tradition and wisdom. Its enduring legacy serves as a testament to the profound impact of nature's remedies on human health and well-being.

Composition and Nutritional Profile

Black seed oil is renowned for its rich and complex composition, which includes a diverse array of bioactive compounds essential for health and well-being. This remarkable oil is a veritable powerhouse of nutrients, boasting a unique blend of fatty acids, vitamins, minerals, and phytochemicals.

Nutritional Profile:

Nutrient	Amount per 3.5 ounces (100g)
Total Fat	3.53 ounces
Saturated Fat	0.53 ounces
Monounsaturated Fat	0.88 ounces
Polyunsaturated Fat	2.12 ounces
Vitamin E	0.28 milligrams (mg)
Thiamine (Vitamin B1)	0.23 milligrams (mg)
Riboflavin (Vitamin B2)	0.07 milligrams (mg)
Niacin (Vitamin B3)	0.35 milligrams (mg)
Calcium	17.7 milligrams (mg)
Iron	0.35 milligrams (mg)
Magnesium	17.7 milligrams (mg)
Phosphorus	35.5 milligrams (mg)
Zinc	0.35 milligrams (mg)

Key Components:

- Fatty Acids: Essential for cellular function and energy production, the fatty acids in black seed oil include saturated, monounsaturated, and polyunsaturated fats.
- Vitamin E: A potent antioxidant that protects cells from damage caused by free radicals and supports immune function.
- B Vitamins (Thiamine, Riboflavin, Niacin): Essential for metabolism, energy production, and nervous system health.
- Minerals (Calcium, Iron, Magnesium, Phosphorus, Zinc): Vital for various bodily functions, including bone health, oxygen transport, muscle function, and immune support.

This comprehensive nutritional profile underscores the extraordinary health benefits of black seed oil and highlights its potential as a valuable addition to a balanced diet and wellness regimen. As we delve deeper into the following chapters, we will explore how each of these components contributes to the remarkable healing properties of black seed oil.

Extraction Methods

The process of extracting black seed oil is a crucial step in preserving its potency and purity, ensuring that the final product retains its therapeutic properties. Various extraction methods are employed to obtain black seed oil, each with its own advantages and considerations.

Extraction Steps:

1. Seed Selection: High-quality black seed oil begins with carefully selecting premium-quality Nigella sativa seeds, free from impurities and contaminants.
2. Cleaning: The seeds are thoroughly cleaned to remove any debris, dust, or foreign particles that may affect the quality of the oil.
3. Grinding: The cleaned seeds are then ground into a fine powder using specialized equipment, increasing the surface area for oil extraction.
4. Pressing: The ground seeds are subjected to mechanical pressing, where pressure is applied to extract the oil from the seed particles.
5. Filtration: The extracted oil undergoes filtration to remove any remaining solids or impurities, resulting in a clear and pure oil.
6. Decanting: In some cases, the oil may undergo a decanting process to separate it from any water or sediment that may have accumulated during extraction.
7. Storage: The final step involves storing the extracted oil in airtight containers away from light and heat to maintain its freshness and potency.

These extraction methods are designed to preserve the integrity of black seed oil, ensuring that it remains a potent and effective natural remedy for various health concerns. As we explore the benefits of black seed oil further in the following chapters, we will delve into the importance of extraction methods and their impact on the quality of the final product.

Quality Considerations: Choosing the Right Product

Selecting the right black seed oil product is paramount to ensuring optimal results and reaping the full benefits of this potent natural remedy. With a myriad of options available in the market, it's essential to be discerning and mindful of certain quality considerations.

Key Considerations:

- **Purity:** Look for black seed oil products that are 100% pure and free from additives, fillers, or preservatives. Pure black seed oil ensures that you're getting the full spectrum of therapeutic compounds without any dilution or contamination.
- **Organic Certification:** Opt for organic-certified black seed oil to ensure that it has been produced without the use of synthetic pesticides, herbicides, or fertilizers. Organic certification guarantees a higher standard of purity and environmental sustainability.
- **Extraction Method:** Consider the extraction method used to produce the black seed oil. Cold-pressed extraction is preferred as it preserves the oil's natural integrity and bioactive compounds, whereas solvent extraction methods may compromise quality.
- **Packaging:** Pay attention to the packaging of the black seed oil product. Choose dark glass bottles or opaque containers to protect the oil from light exposure, which can degrade its quality over time.

- **Transparency:** Seek out brands that provide transparency regarding their sourcing, production methods, and quality testing protocols. Look for products that undergo third-party testing for purity and potency to ensure reliability and efficacy.
- **Storage Instructions:** Check the storage instructions provided by the manufacturer. Proper storage conditions, such as storing the oil in a cool, dark place away from heat and sunlight, are essential for maintaining its freshness and potency.
- **Customer Reviews:** Take into account feedback and reviews from other customers who have used the product. Positive reviews and testimonials can provide valuable insights into the product's effectiveness and quality.

By considering these key factors when choosing a black seed oil product, you can ensure that you're investing in a high-quality supplement that delivers the maximum benefits for your health and well-being. As we delve deeper into the following chapters, we will explore how to incorporate black seed oil into your daily routine effectively.

Health Benefits of Black Seed Oil

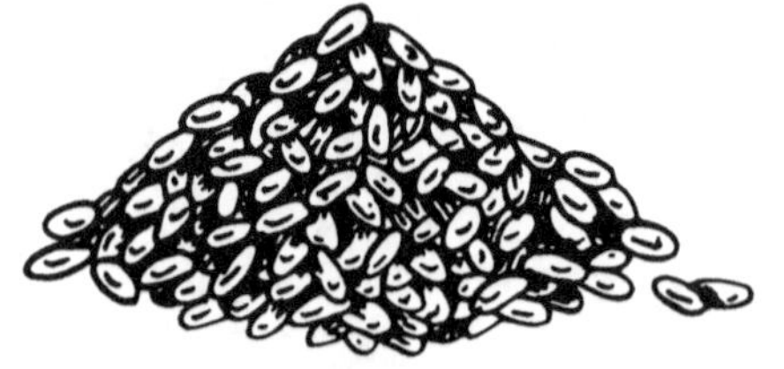

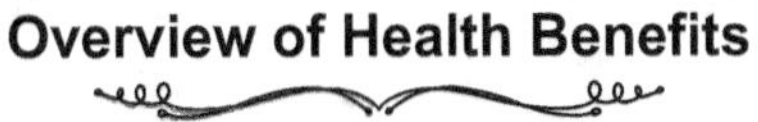

Overview of Health Benefits

Prepare to embark on a journey into the realm of wellness, where the remarkable properties of black seed oil await to transform your health and vitality. Black seed oil, derived from the seeds of the Nigella sativa plant, has long been revered for its myriad health benefits, spanning centuries of traditional use and modern scientific inquiry.

Key Health Benefits:

- **Anti-inflammatory Properties:** Black seed oil exhibits potent anti-inflammatory effects, which can help alleviate symptoms of inflammatory conditions such as arthritis, asthma, and inflammatory bowel disease.
- **Antioxidant Effects:** Rich in antioxidants, black seed oil helps neutralize harmful free radicals in the body, protecting against oxidative stress and cellular damage associated with aging and chronic disease.
- **Immunomodulatory Effects:** Black seed oil has been shown to modulate the immune system, enhancing its ability to defend against infections while also regulating immune responses in autoimmune conditions.
- **Potential for Disease Prevention:** Preliminary research suggests that black seed oil may offer protective effects against a range of diseases, including cancer, cardiovascular disease, and neurodegenerative disorders.
- **Scientific Evidence and Research Studies:** Numerous scientific studies have explored the health benefits of black seed oil, providing compelling evidence of its efficacy in promoting overall health and well-being.

As we delve deeper into the following chapters, we will explore each of these health benefits in greater detail, uncovering the mechanisms behind black seed oil's therapeutic effects and examining the scientific evidence supporting its use as a natural remedy for a wide range of health conditions. Prepare to be enlightened as we unravel the secrets of black seed oil's profound impact on human health.

Anti-inflammatory Properties

Black seed oil possesses potent anti-inflammatory properties attributed to its rich composition of bioactive compounds, particularly thymoquinone. Thymoquinone is a key component of black seed oil that has been extensively studied for its ability to modulate inflammatory pathways within the body.

At a molecular level, thymoquinone exerts its anti-inflammatory effects by inhibiting the production of pro-inflammatory cytokines, enzymes, and mediators involved in the inflammatory response. This includes reducing the expression of nuclear factor-kappa B (NF-kB), a transcription factor that regulates the expression of genes involved in inflammation.

Furthermore, black seed oil has been shown to downregulate the activity of cyclooxygenase-2 (COX-2), an enzyme responsible for the production of inflammatory prostaglandins. By inhibiting COX-2 activity, black seed oil helps mitigate inflammation and alleviate symptoms associated with inflammatory conditions such as arthritis, asthma, and inflammatory bowel disease.

In addition to its direct effects on inflammatory mediators, black seed oil also exhibits antioxidant properties that contribute to its anti-inflammatory effects. By scavenging free radicals and reducing oxidative stress, black seed oil helps protect against inflammation-induced tissue damage and promotes overall health and well-being.

The anti-inflammatory properties of black seed oil have been validated in numerous preclinical and clinical studies, highlighting its potential as a natural remedy for managing inflammatory disorders and supporting overall health.

Sources:

- *Salem, M. L. (2005). Immunomodulatory and therapeutic properties of the Nigella sativa L. seed. International Immunopharmacology, 5(13–14), 1749–1770. doi: 10.1016/j.intimp.2005.06.008*
- *Ahmad, A., Husain, A., Mujeeb, M., Khan, S. A., Najmi, A. K., Siddique, N. A., … Anwar, F. (2013). A review on therapeutic potential of Nigella sativa: A miracle herb. Asian Pacific Journal of Tropical Biomedicine, 3(5), 337–352. doi: 10.1016/S2221-1691(13)60075-1*

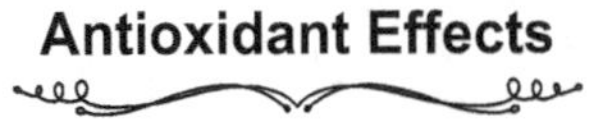

Antioxidant Effects

Black seed oil exhibits remarkable antioxidant effects attributed to its rich content of bioactive compounds, including thymoquinone, thymohydroquinone, and nigellone. These compounds possess potent free radical-scavenging properties, allowing them to neutralize oxidative stress and prevent cellular damage caused by reactive oxygen species (ROS).

At a molecular level, thymoquinone, the predominant active ingredient in black seed oil, functions as a direct antioxidant by donating electrons to unstable free radicals, thereby stabilizing them and preventing them from initiating harmful chain reactions within cells. Thymohydroquinone, another component of black seed oil, enhances the antioxidant activity of thymoquinone by synergistically scavenging free radicals and bolstering cellular defense mechanisms against oxidative stress.

Furthermore, nigellone, a quinone derivative found in black seed oil, contributes to its antioxidant effects by inhibiting the activity of enzymes involved in the production of reactive oxygen species, such as xanthine oxidase and lipoxygenase.

The antioxidant effects of black seed oil extend beyond mere scavenging of free radicals to encompass broader protective effects against oxidative damage to cellular components, including lipids, proteins, and DNA. By reducing oxidative stress and preserving cellular integrity, black seed oil helps mitigate the risk of chronic diseases associated with oxidative damage, such as cardiovascular disease, neurodegenerative disorders, and cancer. Clinical studies have corroborated the antioxidant properties of black seed oil, underscoring its potential as a natural therapeutic agent for promoting overall health and longevity.

Sources:

- *Kanter, M., & Coskun, O. (2006). Antioxidant capacity of nigella sativa (black cumin) seeds. Grasas y Aceites, 57(2), 86–90. doi: 10.3989/gya.2006.v57.i2.47*
- *Mansour, M. A., Nagi, M. N., El-Khatib, A. S., & Al-Bekairi, A. M. (2002). Effects of thymoquinone on antioxidant enzyme activities, lipid peroxidation and DT-diaphorase in different tissues of mice: a possible mechanism of action. Cell Biochemistry and Function, 20(2), 143–151. doi: 10.1002/cbf.942*

Immunomodulatory Effects

Black seed oil exerts profound immunomodulatory effects, influencing the activity and function of the immune system in a manner that promotes overall health and resilience. The immunomodulatory properties of black seed oil are mediated by its bioactive constituents, particularly thymoquinone and nigellone, which interact with various immune cells and signaling pathways. Thymoquinone, the primary active component of black seed oil, has been shown to modulate immune responses by regulating the production of cytokines, chemical messengers that coordinate immune cell activity. Thymoquinone exhibits both immunostimulatory and immunosuppressive effects, depending on the context of immune activation, making it a versatile regulator of immune function.

Additionally, black seed oil has been found to enhance the activity of natural killer (NK) cells, a type of immune cell that plays a crucial role in the body's defense against viruses and cancer cells. By boosting NK cell activity, black seed oil helps bolster the body's innate immune response and enhance its ability to fight off infections and malignancies.

Furthermore, black seed oil has been shown to modulate the balance between Th1 and Th2 immune responses, two distinct arms of the adaptive immune system involved in host defense and allergic reactions, respectively. By promoting a balanced immune response, black seed oil helps maintain immune homeostasis and reduce the risk of autoimmune disorders and allergic diseases. Clinical studies have demonstrated the immunomodulatory effects of black seed oil in various experimental models and human subjects, highlighting its potential as a natural remedy for enhancing immune function and supporting overall health.

Sources:

- *Butt, M. S., Sultan, M. T., Butt, M. S., & Iqbal, J. (2009). Nigella sativa: Reduces the risk of various maladies. Critical Reviews in Food Science and Nutrition, 50(7), 654–665. doi: 10.1080/10408390802427792*
- *Salem, M. L. (2005). Immunomodulatory and therapeutic properties of the Nigella sativa L. seed. International Immunopharmacology, 5(13–14), 1749–1770. doi: 10.1016/j.intimp.2005.06.008*

Potential for Disease Prevention

Black seed oil harbors immense potential for disease prevention, owing to its multifaceted pharmacological properties and diverse array of bioactive compounds. Extensive research has elucidated its role in mitigating the risk of various diseases, encompassing both chronic conditions and acute illnesses.

One of the primary mechanisms through which black seed oil confers protection against disease is its ability to modulate inflammatory pathways within the body. Chronic inflammation is a hallmark of many diseases, including cardiovascular disease, diabetes, and cancer. By exerting anti-inflammatory effects, black seed oil helps reduce inflammation-induced tissue damage and lowers the risk of developing these chronic conditions.

Moreover, black seed oil's antioxidant properties play a pivotal role in disease prevention by neutralizing free radicals and oxidative stress, which are implicated in the pathogenesis of numerous diseases, including neurodegenerative disorders and age-related degenerative conditions. By scavenging free radicals and enhancing cellular defense mechanisms, black seed oil helps safeguard against oxidative damage and promotes overall health and longevity.

Furthermore, black seed oil's immunomodulatory effects contribute to its disease-preventive potential by enhancing immune function and resilience against infections. A robust immune system is essential for combating pathogens and maintaining health, and black seed oil's ability to modulate immune responses helps bolster the body's natural defenses against microbial invaders.

Clinical studies and epidemiological evidence support the disease-preventive properties of black seed oil, underscoring its potential as a valuable adjunct to conventional preventive strategies and a promising avenue for future research into preventive medicine.

Sources:

- *Ahmad, A., Husain, A., Mujeeb, M., Khan, S. A., Najmi, A. K., Siddique, N. A., … Anwar, F. (2013). A review on therapeutic potential of Nigella sativa: A miracle herb. Asian Pacific Journal of Tropical Biomedicine, 3(5), 337–352. doi: 10.1016/S2221-1691(13)60075-1*
- *Gholamnezhad, Z., & Boskabady, M. H. (2019). Hosseini M, khazdair MR, Hosseinifard SM, Rezaee R. The effect of Nigella sativa on inflammation-induced myocardial fibrosis in male rats. Journal of Traditional and Complementary Medicine, 9(4), 310-316. doi: 10.1016/j.jtcme.2018.12.006*

Scientific Evidence and Research Studies

The health benefits attributed to black seed oil are supported by a wealth of scientific evidence derived from preclinical and clinical studies, providing valuable insights into its therapeutic potential and mechanisms of action.

Preclinical studies, conducted primarily in cell culture and animal models, have elucidated the pharmacological properties of black seed oil and its bioactive constituents. These studies have demonstrated black seed oil's anti-inflammatory, antioxidant, immunomodulatory, and anticancer effects, shedding light on the molecular pathways involved in its therapeutic actions.

For example, research has shown that thymoquinone, the main active compound in black seed oil, exerts anti-inflammatory effects by inhibiting the expression of pro-inflammatory cytokines and enzymes, such as interleukin-6 (IL-6) and cyclooxygenase-2 (COX-2). Additionally, thymoquinone's antioxidant properties have been demonstrated through its ability to scavenge free radicals and prevent oxidative damage to cellular components.

Clinical studies involving human participants have further corroborated the health benefits of black seed oil, providing evidence of its efficacy in managing various health conditions. These studies have investigated the use of black seed oil in conditions such as asthma, allergies, diabetes, hypertension, and inflammatory disorders, demonstrating its potential as a safe and effective therapeutic agent.

Furthermore, systematic reviews and meta-analyses have synthesized the findings of multiple studies to evaluate the overall efficacy and safety of black seed oil for specific health outcomes.

These analyses have provided valuable insights into the strength of the evidence supporting the use of black seed oil in clinical practice, guiding healthcare professionals and consumers in making informed decisions about its utilization.

Overall, the scientific evidence supporting the health benefits of black seed oil is robust and continues to grow, highlighting its potential as a valuable adjunct to conventional medical therapies and a promising avenue for future research into natural remedies for health promotion and disease prevention.

Sources:

- *Chehl, N., Chipitsyna, G., Gong, Q., Yeo, C. J., & Arafat, H. A. (2009). Anti-inflammatory effects of the Nigella sativa seed extract, thymoquinone, in pancreatic cancer cells. HPB : The Official Journal of the International Hepato Pancreato Biliary Association, 11(5), 373–381. doi: 10.1111/j.1477-2574.2009.00056.x*
- *Salem, M. L. (2005). Immunomodulatory and therapeutic properties of the Nigella sativa L. seed. International Immunopharmacology, 5(13–14), 1749–1770. doi: 10.1016/j.intimp.2005.06.008*

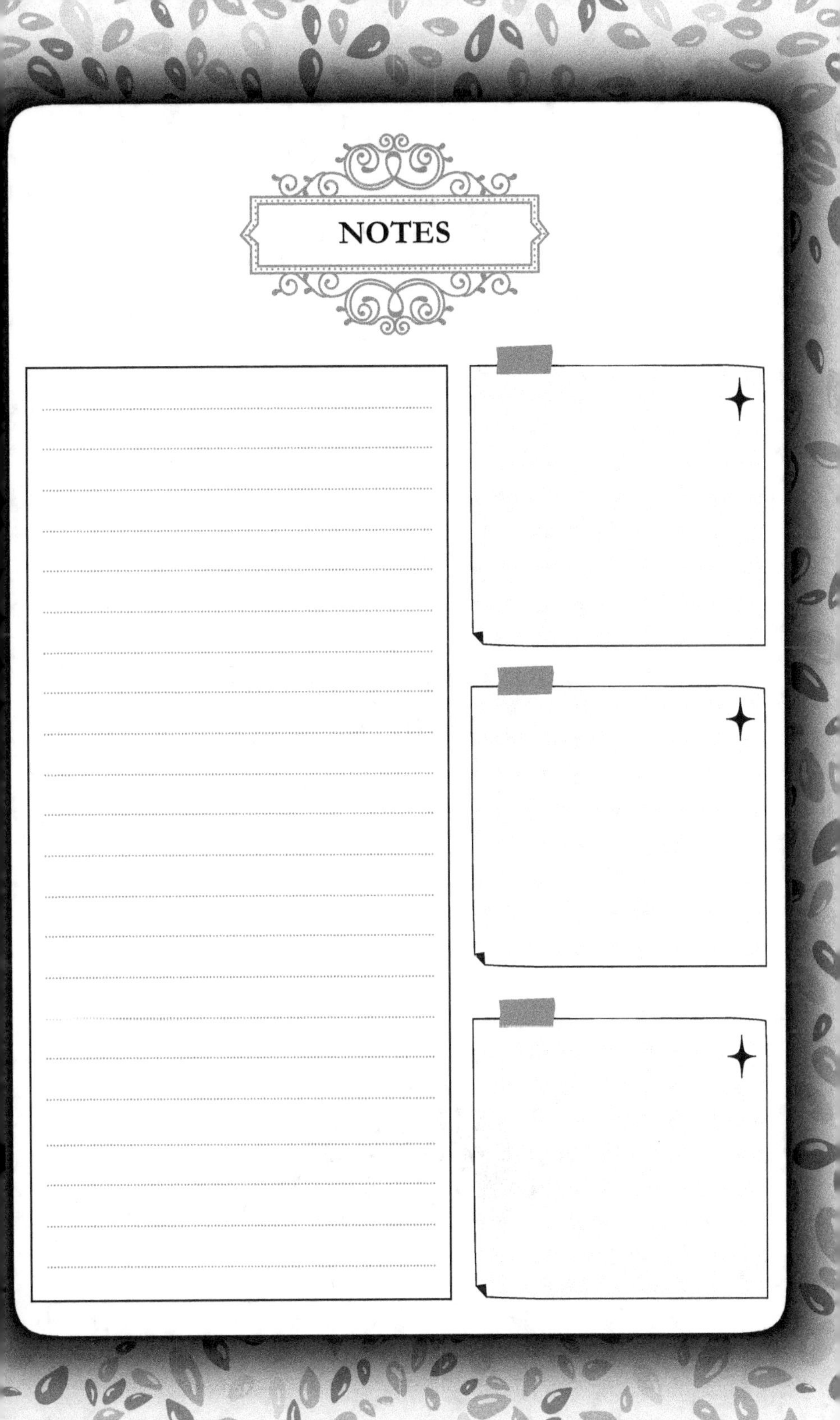

NOTES

Incorporating Black Seed Oil into Daily Routine

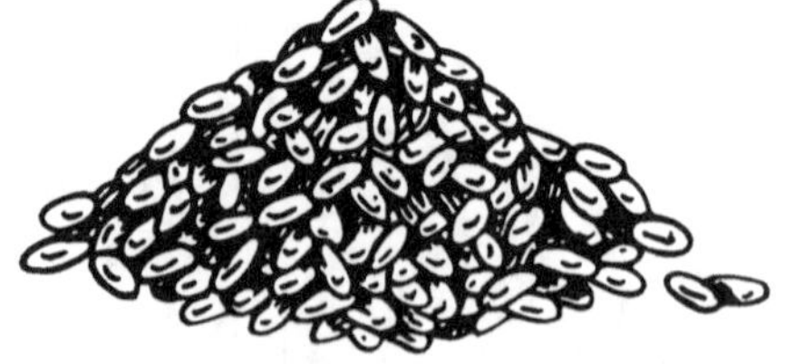

Different Forms of Consumption (capsules, oil, powder)

Incorporating black seed oil into your daily routine offers a convenient and effective way to harness its myriad health benefits. Black seed oil is available in various forms of consumption, each offering unique advantages and considerations. Understanding these different forms can help you choose the most suitable option for integrating black seed oil into your lifestyle.

Forms of Consumption:

- **Capsules:** Black seed oil capsules provide a convenient and standardized way to consume the oil. Encapsulating the oil ensures precise dosing and eliminates the need for measuring or handling liquid oil. Capsules also offer portability and ease of administration, making them ideal for individuals on the go or those who prefer a hassle-free supplement regimen.
- **Oil:** Pure black seed oil is available in liquid form, allowing for versatile and customizable dosing. Liquid oil can be consumed orally by swallowing directly or mixing with food or beverages. It can also be applied topically to the skin or hair for therapeutic purposes. Liquid oil offers flexibility in dosing and application, making it suitable for individuals seeking personalized wellness solutions.
- **Powder:** Black seed oil powder is a convenient option for those who prefer alternative forms of consumption. Powdered oil is typically encapsulated or mixed with other ingredients to create supplements or functional food products. Powdered formulations may offer enhanced stability and shelf life compared to liquid oil, making them suitable for long-term storage and travel.

ISelecting the most suitable form of black seed oil consumption depends on individual preferences, lifestyle factors, and therapeutic goals. Whether you prefer the convenience of capsules, the versatility of liquid oil, or the innovation of powdered formulations, incorporating black seed oil into your daily routine can support your journey towards optimal health and well-being. Experimenting with different forms of consumption allows you to discover the most effective and enjoyable way to experience the benefits of black seed oil, empowering you to take control of your health and vitality.

Dosage Guidelines

Determining the appropriate dosage of black seed oil is essential for optimizing its therapeutic benefits while minimizing the risk of adverse effects. Dosage guidelines for black seed oil vary depending on factors such as age, health status, and specific health goals. Understanding these guidelines can help individuals achieve safe and effective supplementation with black seed oil.

Key Considerations:

- **Individual Factors:** The optimal dosage of black seed oil may vary depending on individual factors such as age, weight, overall health status, and the presence of any underlying medical conditions. It is advisable to consult with a healthcare professional to determine the most appropriate dosage for your specific needs.
- **Health Goals:** The dosage of black seed oil may also be influenced by the specific health goals or conditions being targeted. For general health maintenance, lower doses may be sufficient, while higher doses may be recommended for therapeutic purposes or to address specific health concerns.
- **Formulation Strength:** The concentration of active ingredients in black seed oil formulations can vary between products. It is important to carefully read product labels and follow manufacturer recommendations regarding dosage instructions. Higher concentration formulations may require smaller doses to achieve desired effects.

- **Gradual Titration:** When starting black seed oil supplementation, it is advisable to begin with a lower dose and gradually titrate upwards as tolerated. This approach allows the body to acclimate to the supplement and helps minimize the risk of digestive discomfort or other adverse reactions.
- Clinical Evidence: While there is limited clinical evidence to establish standardized dosage guidelines for black seed oil, anecdotal reports and traditional usage suggest that typical doses range from 500 mg to 2,000 mg per day for adults. However, individual responses to supplementation may vary, and it is important to start with a conservative dose and adjust as needed based on personal tolerance and response.

Determining the optimal dosage of black seed oil requires careful consideration of individual factors, health goals, and product formulations. By consulting with a healthcare professional and following recommended dosage guidelines, individuals can safely and effectively incorporate black seed oil into their daily routine to support overall health and well-being.

As with any supplement, it is important to monitor for any potential side effects or interactions with other medications and discontinue use if any adverse reactions occur. With responsible supplementation, black seed oil can be a valuable addition to a holistic approach to health and wellness.

Potential Side Effects and Precautions

Incorporating black seed oil into your daily routine can offer numerous health benefits, but it's important to be aware of potential side effects and take necessary precautions to ensure safe usage. While black seed oil is generally considered safe for most individuals when used appropriately, some people may experience adverse reactions or interactions under certain circumstances.

Common Side Effects:

- **Digestive Discomfort:** Some individuals may experience mild gastrointestinal discomfort, such as nausea, bloating, or diarrhea, particularly when starting black seed oil supplementation or using higher doses. These symptoms are usually transient and tend to resolve on their own as the body adjusts to the supplement.
- **Allergic Reactions:** Although rare, allergic reactions to black seed oil have been reported in some individuals. Symptoms of an allergic reaction may include skin rash, itching, swelling, or difficulty breathing. If you experience any signs of an allergic reaction after using black seed oil, discontinue use immediately and seek medical attention.

Precautions:

- **Pregnancy and Breastfeeding:** Pregnant or breastfeeding women should exercise caution when using black seed oil, as its safety during pregnancy and lactation has not been fully established. Consult with a healthcare professional before using black seed oil if you are pregnant, nursing, or planning to become pregnant.
- **Medical Conditions:** Individuals with certain medical conditions, such as bleeding disorders, diabetes, or autoimmune diseases, should consult with a healthcare provider before using black seed oil, as it may interact with medications or exacerbate underlying health issues.
- **Drug Interactions:** Black seed oil may interact with certain medications, including blood thinners, antidiabetic drugs, and immunosuppressants. If you are taking any medications, discuss with your healthcare provider before starting black seed oil supplementation to avoid potential interactions.

While black seed oil offers promising health benefits, it's important to approach its use with caution and awareness of potential side effects and precautions. By following recommended dosage guidelines, monitoring for any adverse reactions, and consulting with a healthcare professional when needed, you can safely incorporate black seed oil into your daily routine to support your health and well-being.

If you experience any concerning symptoms or have questions about black seed oil supplementation, don't hesitate to seek guidance from a qualified healthcare provider. With responsible use and informed decision-making, you can enjoy the potential benefits of black seed oil while minimizing the risk of adverse effects.

Interactions with Medications

Incorporating black seed oil into your daily routine can provide various health benefits, but it's essential to be aware of potential interactions with medications to ensure safe and effective use. While black seed oil is generally considered safe when used appropriately, it may interact with certain medications, leading to adverse effects or reduced efficacy.

Understanding Interactions:

- **Blood Thinners:** Black seed oil may have mild anticoagulant effects, which could potentially interact with medications such as warfarin (Coumadin) or aspirin. Concurrent use of black seed oil with blood thinners may increase the risk of bleeding or bruising. It is advisable to monitor closely if using both black seed oil and blood thinners concurrently and consult with a healthcare professional for appropriate dosage adjustments.
- **Antidiabetic Drugs:** Black seed oil may lower blood sugar levels, which could enhance the effects of antidiabetic medications such as insulin or oral hypoglycemic agents. Individuals taking medications for diabetes should monitor their blood sugar levels closely when using black seed oil and consult with a healthcare provider for adjustments in medication dosage as needed.
- **Immunosuppressants:** Black seed oil has immunomodulatory properties that could potentially interact with immunosuppressant medications, such as corticosteroids or cyclosporine. Concurrent use may alter immune function and affect the efficacy of immunosuppressive therapy. It is advisable to consult with a healthcare provider before using

black seed oil if taking immunosuppressants.

Precautions:

- **Consultation with Healthcare Provider:** Before starting black seed oil supplementation, it is essential to inform your healthcare provider about all medications you are currently taking, including prescription drugs, over-the-counter medications, and dietary supplements. Your healthcare provider can assess potential interactions and provide guidance on safe and appropriate use.
- **Monitoring:** If using black seed oil alongside medications, it is crucial to monitor for any signs of adverse effects or changes in medication efficacy. Regular monitoring of relevant health parameters, such as blood sugar levels or clotting times, can help detect and manage any potential interactions effectively.

While black seed oil offers promising health benefits, it's important to exercise caution and awareness of potential interactions with medications. By communicating openly with your healthcare provider, monitoring for any adverse effects, and following recommended dosage guidelines, you can safely incorporate black seed oil into your daily routine to support your health and well-being.

If you have any concerns about potential interactions or need guidance on using black seed oil alongside medications, don't hesitate to consult with a qualified healthcare professional. With informed decision-making and responsible use, you can maximize the benefits of black seed oil while minimizing the risk of adverse interactions with medications.

Tips for Safe Use

Incorporating black seed oil into your daily routine can offer numerous health benefits, but it's essential to use it safely and responsibly. Here are some tips to ensure safe and effective use of black seed oil:

Consult with a Healthcare Professional: Before starting black seed oil supplementation, consult with a qualified healthcare provider, especially if you have any underlying medical conditions or are taking medications. A healthcare professional can provide personalized guidance and help determine the most appropriate dosage and usage regimen for your individual needs.

Start with a Low Dose: If you are new to black seed oil, start with a low dose and gradually increase it as tolerated. This allows your body to adjust to the supplement and minimizes the risk of potential side effects. Monitor for any adverse reactions and discontinue use if you experience any discomfort.

Choose High-Quality Products: Select black seed oil products from reputable manufacturers known for their quality and purity. Look for products that undergo rigorous testing for potency, purity, and safety. Avoid products that contain additives, fillers, or artificial ingredients.

Follow Dosage Guidelines: Adhere to recommended dosage guidelines provided by the manufacturer or your healthcare provider. Avoid exceeding the recommended dosage unless advised by a healthcare professional. Proper dosing ensures optimal benefits while minimizing the risk of adverse effects.

Store Properly: Store black seed oil in a cool, dry place away from direct sunlight and heat to preserve its freshness and potency. Close the bottle tightly after each use to prevent oxidation and maintain product integrity.

Monitor for Adverse Effects: Pay attention to how your body responds to black seed oil supplementation. Monitor for any adverse effects, such as gastrointestinal discomfort, allergic reactions, or changes in health parameters. If you experience any concerning symptoms, discontinue use and seek medical attention.

Seek Professional Advice: If you have any questions or concerns about using black seed oil, don't hesitate to seek guidance from a qualified healthcare professional. They can provide expert advice, address any concerns, and ensure that black seed oil supplementation aligns with your overall health goals.

NOTES

Black Seed Oil for Natural Skincare and Haircare

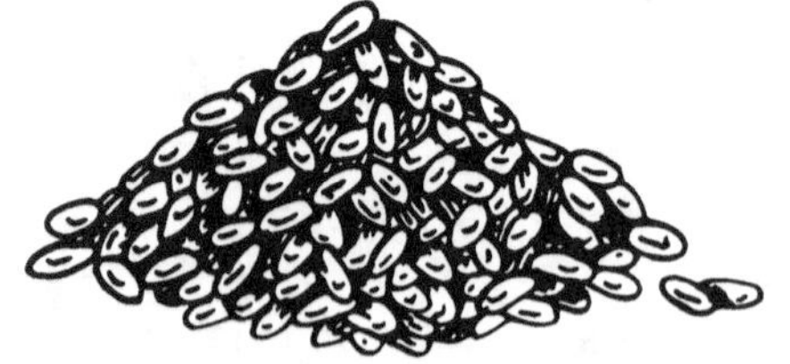

Properties Beneficial for Skin and Hair

Black seed oil, derived from the seeds of the Nigella sativa plant, possesses a plethora of properties that make it a valuable addition to skincare and haircare routines. Rich in essential fatty acids, vitamins, minerals, and antioxidants, black seed oil offers numerous benefits for promoting healthy skin and hair.

Moisturizing:

Black seed oil acts as a natural emollient, helping to lock in moisture and prevent dryness. Its rich lipid content nourishes the skin and hair, leaving them feeling soft, smooth, and hydrated.

Anti-inflammatory:

The anti-inflammatory properties of black seed oil can help soothe irritated skin and reduce redness, swelling, and inflammation associated with conditions such as acne, eczema, and psoriasis. It calms sensitive skin and promotes a more balanced complexion.

Antioxidant:

Black seed oil is rich in antioxidants such as thymoquinone and nigellone, which help neutralize free radicals and protect the skin and hair from oxidative stress and environmental damage. This can help prevent premature aging, including wrinkles, fine lines, and dullness.

Antibacterial and Antifungal:

The antibacterial and antifungal properties of black seed oil make it effective in combating acne-causing bacteria, fungal infections, and other microbial pathogens. It helps cleanse the skin and scalp, reducing the risk of breakouts and dandruff.

Wound Healing:

Black seed oil promotes wound healing and tissue regeneration, making it beneficial for treating cuts, scrapes, burns, and other minor skin injuries. Its anti-inflammatory and antimicrobial properties help prevent infection and accelerate the healing process.

Hair Growth Stimulation:

Black seed oil stimulates hair follicles and promotes healthy hair growth. Its nourishing properties strengthen the hair shaft, reduce breakage and split ends, and improve overall hair texture and thickness. It can also help prevent hair loss and baldness.

Sebum Regulation:

Black seed oil helps balance sebum production in the skin and scalp, making it suitable for all skin and hair types, including oily and acne-prone. It regulates oil production without clogging pores or causing greasiness, promoting a clearer complexion and healthier scalp.

UV Protection:

Black seed oil provides natural protection against UV radiation and sun damage. Its antioxidant properties help shield the skin and hair from harmful UV rays, reducing the risk of sunburn, premature aging, and skin cancer.

Incorporating black seed oil into your skincare and haircare routine can help promote healthy, radiant skin and lustrous hair. Its multifaceted properties make it a versatile and effective natural remedy for addressing various skin and hair concerns, from dryness and inflammation to acne and hair loss.

DIY Skincare and Haircare Recipes

Harnessing the natural benefits of black seed oil, you can create homemade skincare and haircare products that are both effective and gentle on your skin and hair. Here are some simple DIY recipes to incorporate black seed oil into your beauty routine:

1. Nourishing Facial Mask:

- Ingredients:
  - 1 tablespoon black seed oil
  - 1 tablespoon raw honey
  - 1 tablespoon plain yogurt
- Instructions:
  - In a small bowl, mix together black seed oil, raw honey, and plain yogurt until well combined.
  - Apply the mixture to clean, dry skin, avoiding the eye area.
  - Leave the mask on for 15-20 minutes, then rinse thoroughly with warm water.
  - Follow up with your favorite moisturizer for added hydration.

Notes :

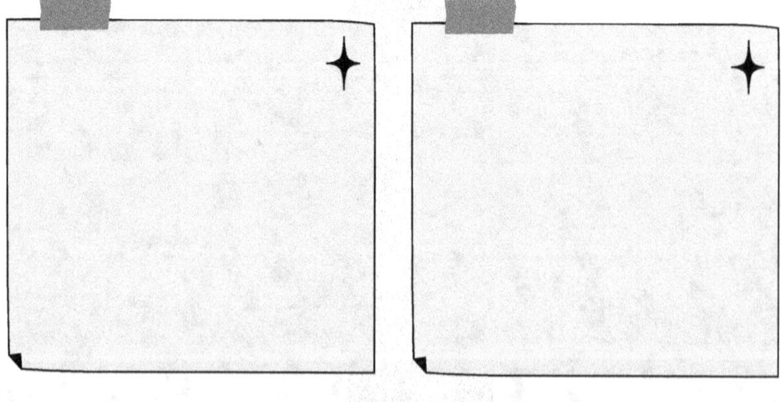

2. Hydrating Hair Mask:

- Ingredients:
    - 2 tablespoons black seed oil
    - 1 ripe avocado
    - 1 tablespoon honey
- Instructions:
    - Mash the avocado in a bowl until smooth.
    - Add black seed oil and honey to the mashed avocado and mix well.
    - Apply the mixture to damp hair, focusing on the ends and any dry or damaged areas.
    - Cover your hair with a shower cap or towel and leave the mask on for 30-60 minutes.
    - Rinse thoroughly with lukewarm water, then shampoo and condition as usual.

Notes :

3. Soothing Body Scrub:

- Ingredients:
    - 1/2 cup granulated sugar
    - 1/4 cup coconut oil
    - 2 tablespoons black seed oil
    - 5-10 drops lavender essential oil (optional)
- Instructions:
    - In a mixing bowl, combine granulated sugar, coconut oil, black seed oil, and lavender essential oil (if using).
    - Mix until all ingredients are well incorporated and the scrub has a uniform texture.
    - Gently massage the scrub onto damp skin in circular motions, focusing on rough areas like elbows, knees, and heels.
    - Rinse off with warm water and pat skin dry. Follow up with a moisturizer for extra hydration.

Notes :

4. Strengthening Hair Serum:

- Ingredients:
  - 2 tablespoons black seed oil
  - 1 tablespoon argan oil
  - 5 drops rosemary essential oil
- Instructions:
  - In a small glass bottle, combine black seed oil, argan oil, and rosemary essential oil.
  - Close the bottle tightly and shake well to mix the ingredients thoroughly.
  - Apply a few drops of the serum to your fingertips and massage into the scalp and hair roots.
  - Use daily as a leave-in treatment to nourish and strengthen the hair follicles.

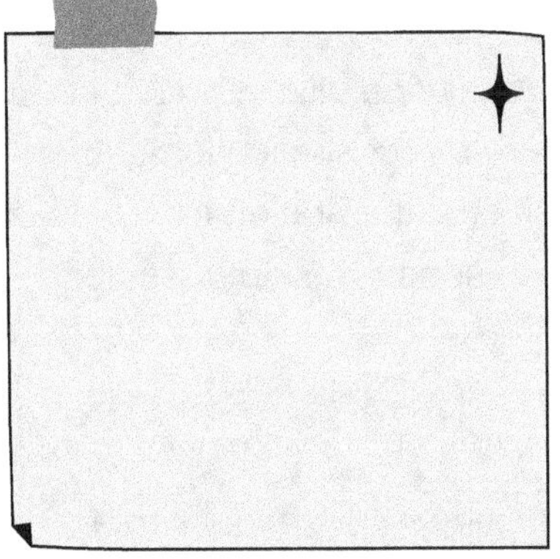

These DIY recipes allow you to customize your skincare and haircare routine while reaping the benefits of black seed oil's natural properties. Experiment with different ingredients and adjust the recipes to suit your preferences and specific skincare or haircare needs.

Tips for Safe Application

Ensuring safe and effective application of black seed oil in your skincare and haircare routine is essential for maximizing its benefits while minimizing the risk of adverse reactions. Here are some tips to help you safely incorporate black seed oil into your beauty regimen:

Patch Test:

Before using black seed oil on larger areas of your skin or scalp, perform a patch test to check for any allergic reactions or sensitivities. Apply a small amount of diluted black seed oil to a discreet area of your skin, such as the inner forearm, and wait 24 hours to observe for any adverse reactions before proceeding with regular use.

Dilution:

Black seed oil is potent and should ideally be diluted with a carrier oil or other skincare ingredients before direct application to the skin or hair. Dilution helps reduce the risk of skin irritation or sensitization, especially for those with sensitive skin or scalp conditions.

Avoid Contact with Eyes:

When applying black seed oil to the skin or hair, avoid contact with the eyes and mucous membranes to prevent irritation or discomfort. If accidental contact occurs, rinse thoroughly with water and seek medical attention if irritation persists.

Sun Protection:

While black seed oil offers some natural protection against UV radiation, it's essential to continue using sunscreen and protective clothing when exposed to the sun for extended periods. Incorporate black seed oil into your skincare routine as an additional protective measure, not as a replacement for sunscreen.

Consultation with a Professional:

Before incorporating black seed oil into your skincare or haircare routine, it's advisable to consult with a qualified skincare specialist, dermatologist, or trichologist, especially if you have existing skin or scalp conditions, allergies, or are pregnant or breastfeeding. A professional can provide personalized advice, dosage recommendations, and guidance tailored to your specific needs and concerns.

Monitor for Adverse Reactions:

Pay attention to how your skin and hair respond to black seed oil application. If you experience any irritation, redness, itching, or other adverse reactions, discontinue use immediately and rinse thoroughly with water. Consult with a healthcare professional if symptoms persist or worsen.

Storage and Shelf Life:

Store black seed oil in a cool, dry place away from direct sunlight and heat to preserve its freshness and potency. Check the expiration date on the packaging and discard any expired or rancid oil to ensure safety and efficacy.

By following these tips for safe application, you can incorporate black seed oil into your skincare and haircare routine with confidence, knowing that you're taking the necessary precautions to protect and nourish your skin and hair effectively. Remember to prioritize safety and consult with a professional for personalized advice and guidance tailored to your individual needs and concerns.

NOTES

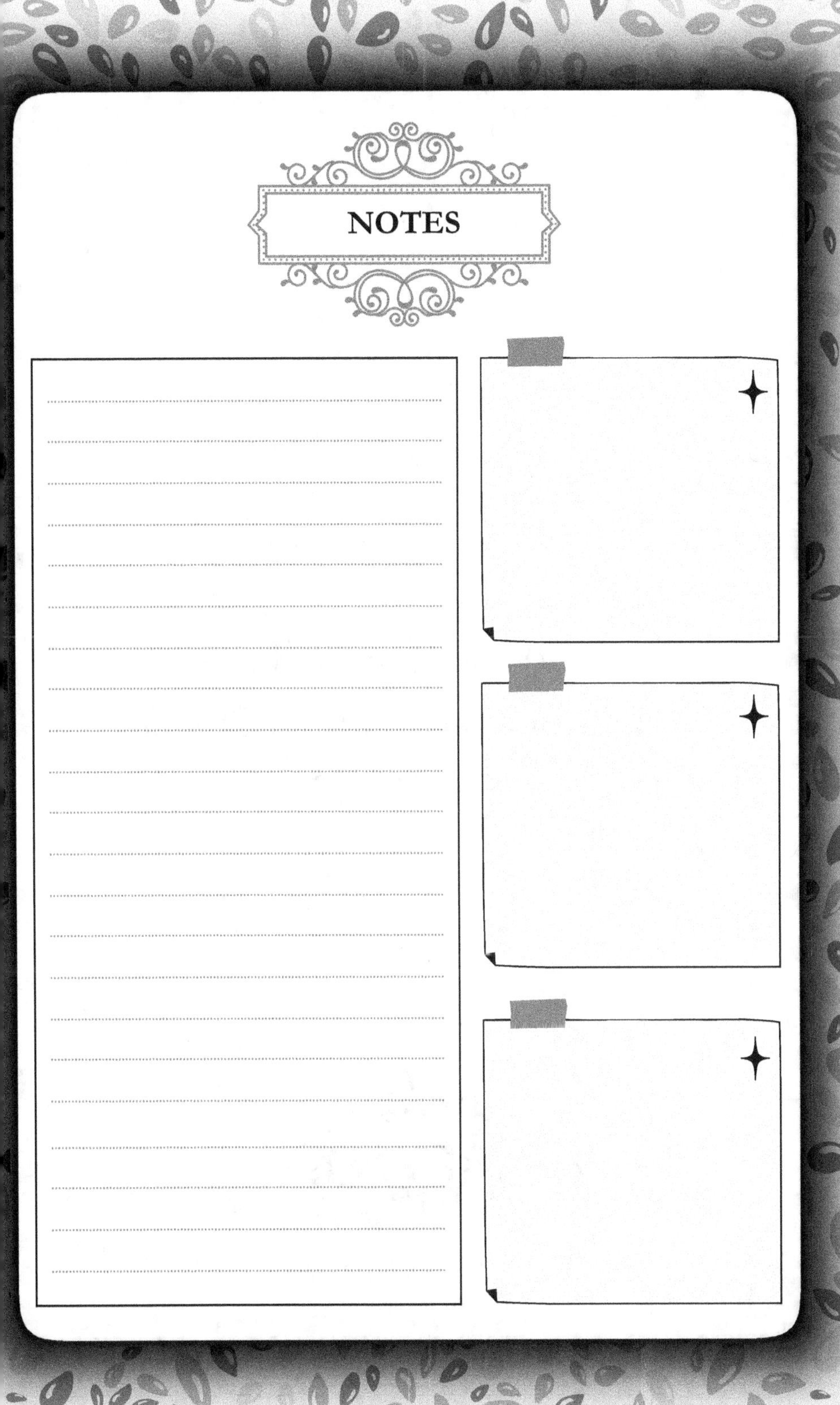

Black Seed Oil in Traditional and Ethnic Cuisine

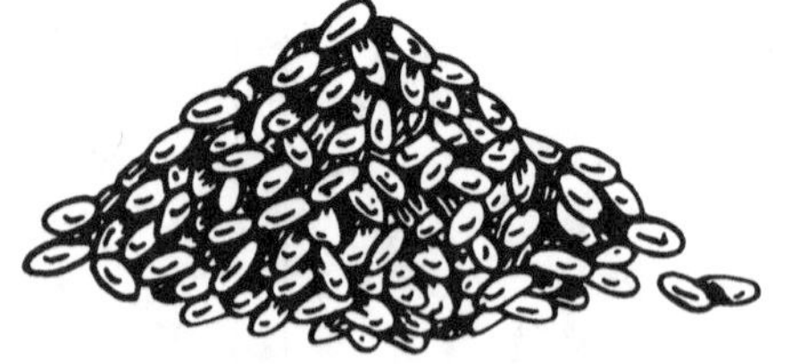

Culinary Uses Across Cultures

Black seed oil, also known as black cumin seed oil or nigella sativa oil, has a rich culinary history spanning various cultures and cuisines around the world. Its distinct flavor and nutritional benefits have made it a staple ingredient in traditional dishes and culinary practices across regions. Here's an overview of the culinary uses of black seed oil across different cultures.

Middle Eastern Cuisine

In Middle Eastern cuisine, particularly in countries like Egypt, Iran, and Turkey, black seed oil is a common ingredient used in both savory and sweet dishes. It is often drizzled over salads, dips, and grilled meats for added flavor and nutritional benefits. Additionally, black seed oil is incorporated into baked goods, pastries, and desserts for its aromatic and earthy taste.

South Asian Cuisine

In South Asian cuisine, black seed oil, known as kalonji oil or kalonji ka tel, is widely used in cooking, especially in Indian and Pakistani cuisines. It is a key ingredient in spice blends such as garam masala and curry powders, adding depth and complexity to dishes. Black seed oil is also used for tempering, where it is heated with spices and added to dishes at the end of cooking to enhance their flavor.

Mediterranean Cuisine

In Mediterranean cuisine, particularly in countries like Greece and Lebanon, black seed oil is used in various traditional recipes, including salads, marinades, and dips. It is prized for its robust flavor and nutritional properties, often paired with fresh herbs, garlic, and lemon juice to create vibrant and aromatic dishes.

African Cuisine

In African cuisine, black seed oil is commonly used in North African and Ethiopian cooking. It is added to soups, stews, and vegetable dishes for its distinctive flavor and health benefits. In Ethiopian cuisine, black seed oil is a key ingredient in traditional spice blends like berbere and mitmita, which are used to season meats and lentil dishes.

Latin American Cuisine

In Latin American cuisine, particularly in countries like Mexico and Colombia, black seed oil is less common but still used in certain regional dishes. It may be incorporated into marinades, sauces, and dressings for its unique flavor profile and potential health benefits.

Overall, black seed oil's versatility and culinary appeal have led to its widespread use in various cuisines worldwide, where it adds depth, aroma, and nutritional value to a wide range of dishes.

Recipes and Cooking Techniques

Incorporating black seed oil into traditional and ethnic cuisine opens up a world of culinary possibilities. Whether used as a finishing oil, a marinade ingredient, or a flavor enhancer, black seed oil can elevate the taste and nutritional value of a wide range of dishes.

Here are some recipes and cooking techniques showcasing the versatility of black seed oil.

Recipes:

- **Black Seed Oil Salad Dressing:**
  - Ingredients:
    - 1/4 cup black seed oil
    - 2 tablespoons apple cider vinegar
    - 1 tablespoon honey
    - 1 teaspoon Dijon mustard
    - Salt and pepper to taste
  - Instructions:
    - In a small bowl, whisk together black seed oil, apple cider vinegar, honey, and Dijon mustard until well combined.
    - Season with salt and pepper to taste.
    - Drizzle the dressing over your favorite salad greens and toss to coat evenly. Serve immediately.

- **Roasted Vegetables with Black Seed Oil:**
  - Ingredients:
    - 2 cups mixed vegetables (such as carrots, bell peppers, zucchini)
    - 2 tablespoons black seed oil
    - 1 teaspoon dried thyme
    - Salt and pepper to taste
  - Instructions:
    - Preheat the oven to 400°F (200°C).
    - In a large bowl, toss the mixed vegetables with black seed oil, dried thyme, salt, and pepper until evenly coated.
    - Spread the vegetables in a single layer on a baking sheet.
    - Roast in the preheated oven for 20-25 minutes, or until the vegetables are tender and lightly browned.
    - Serve hot as a side dish or as a topping for salads or grain bowls.

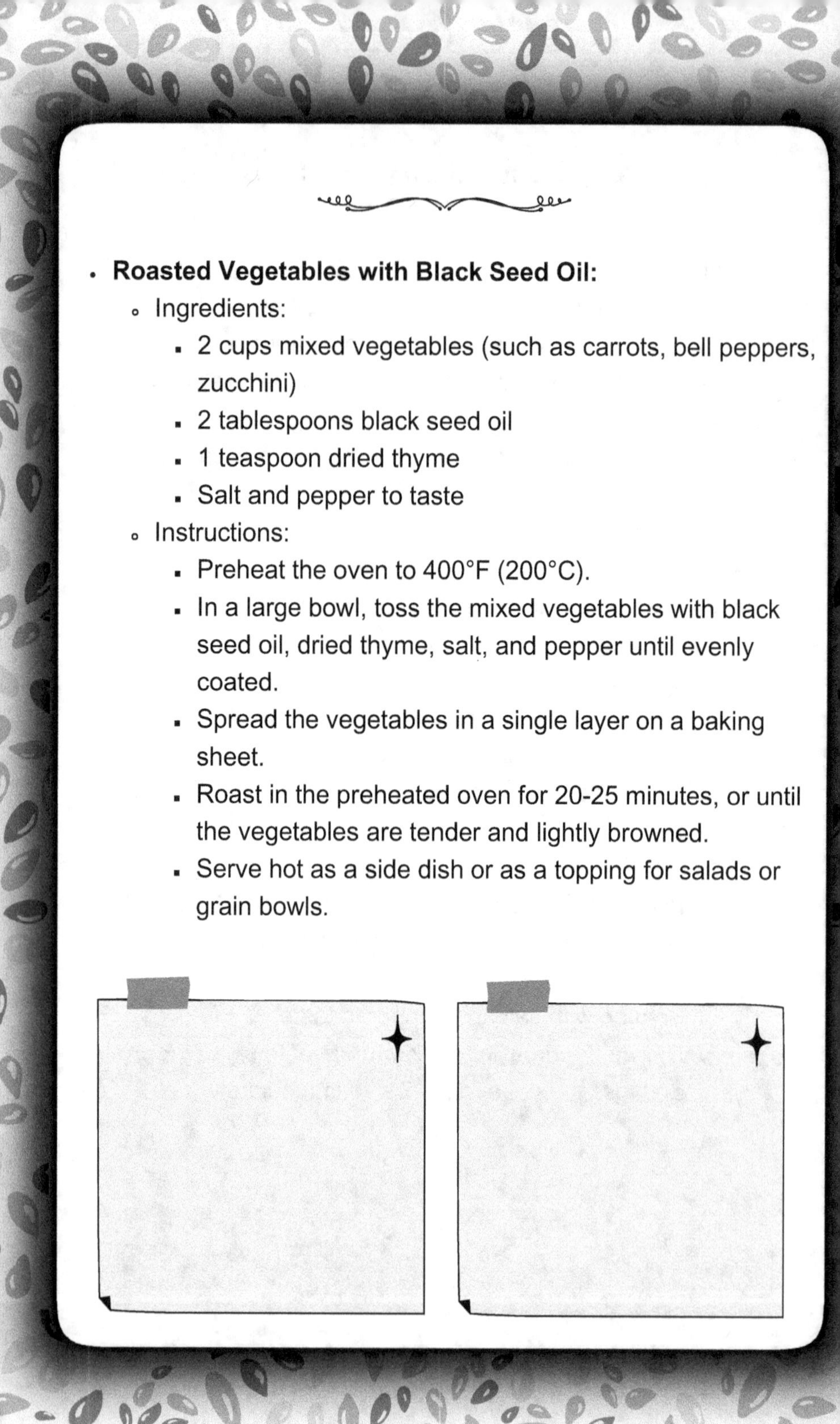

- **Black Seed Oil Hummus:**
  - Ingredients:
    - 1 can (15 ounces) chickpeas, drained and rinsed
    - 3 tablespoons tahini
    - 2 tablespoons black seed oil
    - 2 cloves garlic, minced
    - Juice of 1 lemon
    - Salt to taste
  - Instructions:
    - In a food processor, combine chickpeas, tahini, black seed oil, minced garlic, lemon juice, and salt.
    - Process until smooth and creamy, scraping down the sides of the bowl as needed.
    - If the hummus is too thick, add a tablespoon of water at a time until desired consistency is reached.
    - Transfer the hummus to a serving bowl and drizzle with additional black seed oil before serving. Serve with pita bread, crackers, or fresh vegetables.

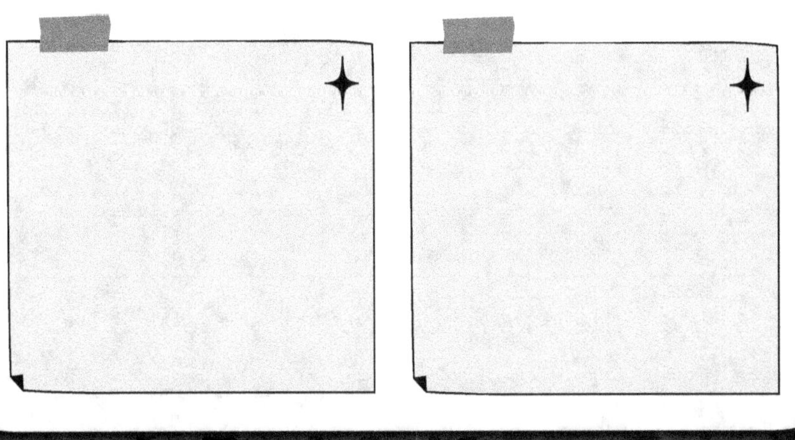

- **Black Seed Oil Roasted Chicken:**
  - Ingredients:
    - 4 bone-in, skin-on chicken thighs
    - 2 tablespoons black seed oil
    - 2 cloves garlic, minced
    - 1 teaspoon ground cumin
    - 1 teaspoon paprika
    - Salt and pepper to taste
  - Instructions:
    - Preheat the oven to 375°F (190°C).
    - In a small bowl, mix together black seed oil, minced garlic, ground cumin, paprika, salt, and pepper.
    - Rub the chicken thighs with the black seed oil mixture, making sure to coat them evenly.
    - Place the chicken thighs on a baking sheet lined with parchment paper.
    - Roast in the preheated oven for 25-30 minutes, or until the chicken is cooked through and golden brown.
    - Serve hot with your favorite side dishes.

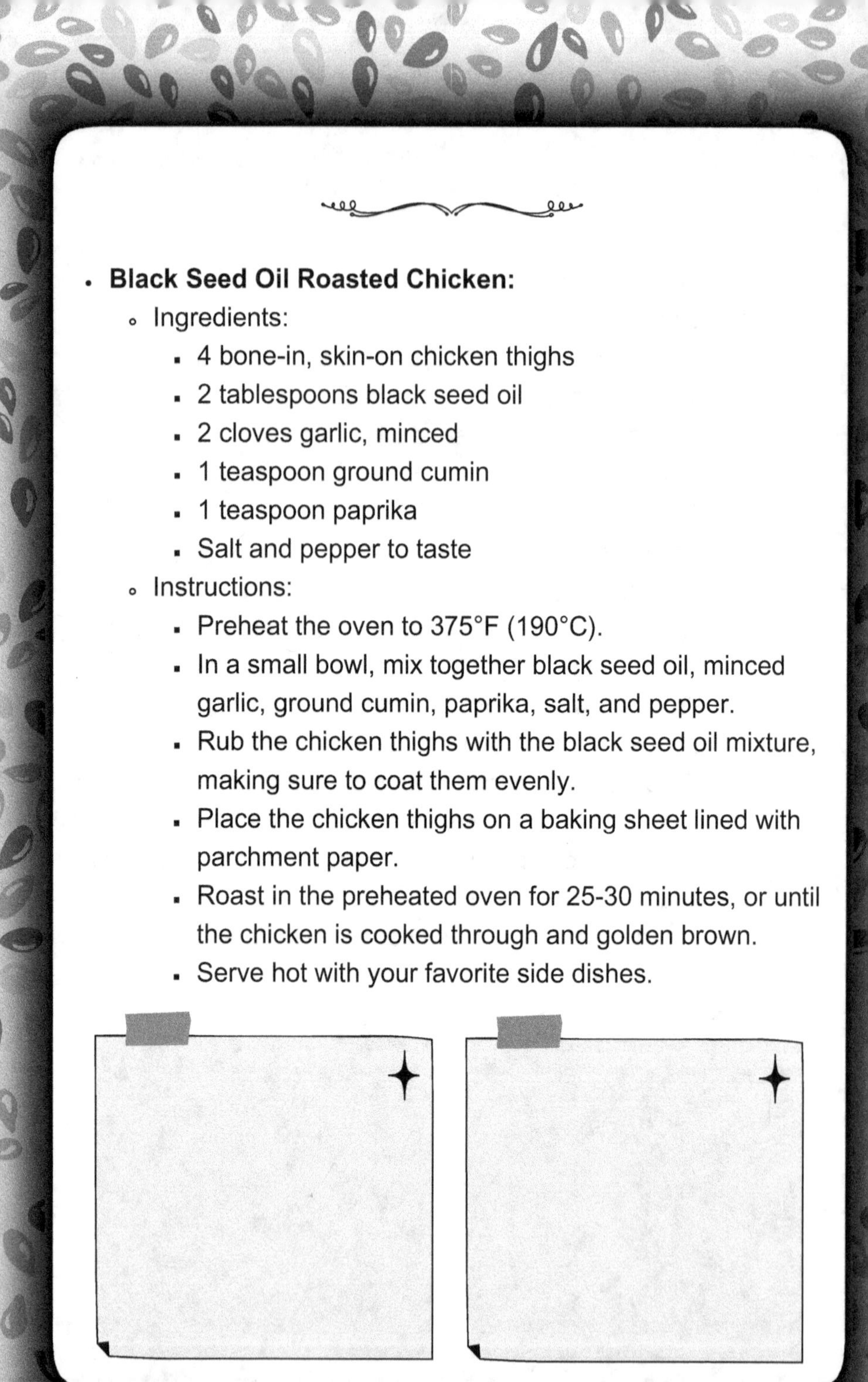

- **Black Seed Oil Smoothie Bowl:**
  - Ingredients:
    - 1 frozen banana
    - 1/2 cup frozen mixed berries
    - 1 tablespoon black seed oil
    - 1/2 cup Greek yogurt
    - 1/4 cup almond milk
    - Toppings: granola, sliced fruit, chia seeds
  - Instructions:
    - In a blender, combine frozen banana, frozen mixed berries, black seed oil, Greek yogurt, and almond milk.
    - Blend until smooth and creamy, adding more almond milk if needed to reach desired consistency.
    - Pour the smoothie into a bowl and top with granola, sliced fruit, and chia seeds.
    - Drizzle with an additional swirl of black seed oil before serving for added flavor and nutritional benefits.

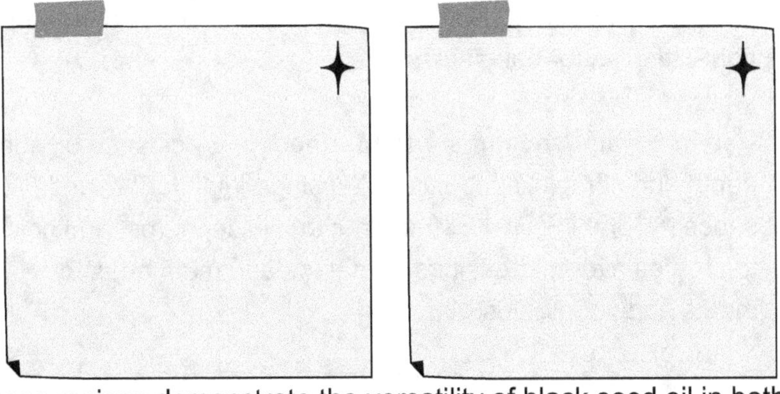

These recipes demonstrate the versatility of black seed oil in both savory and sweet dishes, highlighting its unique flavor profile and nutritional properties.

Culinary Tips and Tricks

Mastering the use of black seed oil in traditional and ethnic cuisine requires an understanding of its unique characteristics and culinary applications. Here are some expert tips and tricks to help you make the most out of black seed oil in your cooking:

- **Use as a Finishing Oil:** Black seed oil is best used as a finishing oil rather than for high-heat cooking. Drizzle it over cooked dishes just before serving to preserve its delicate flavor and maximize its nutritional benefits.

- **Pair with Complementary Flavors:** Experiment with different flavor combinations to enhance the taste of your dishes. Pair black seed oil with ingredients like lemon, garlic, herbs, and spices to create harmonious flavor profiles.

- **Store Properly**: Store black seed oil in a cool, dark place away from direct sunlight to prevent oxidation and preserve its freshness. Consider transferring it to a dark glass bottle with a tight-fitting lid for optimal storage.

- **Use in Salad Dressings and Marinades**: Black seed oil adds depth and complexity to salad dressings, marinades, and sauces. Combine it with vinegar, citrus juice, herbs, and spices to create flavorful dressings for salads and marinades for meats and vegetables.

- **Experiment with Different Cuisines:** Incorporate black seed oil into a variety of cuisines to explore its versatility. From Middle Eastern and South Asian dishes to Mediterranean and Latin American recipes, black seed oil can complement a wide range of culinary traditions.

- **Start with Small Amounts:** Since black seed oil has a strong flavor, start with small amounts and adjust to taste. A little goes a long way, so use it sparingly to avoid overpowering other flavors in your dishes.

- **Enhance Baked Goods:** Add a unique twist to baked goods by incorporating black seed oil into recipes for bread, muffins, cakes, and cookies. Its nutty flavor and nutritional properties can elevate the taste and texture of your baked treats.

- **Combine with Nut Butters:** Mix black seed oil with nut butters like almond butter or tahini to create flavorful spreads for toast, sandwiches, or fruit. The combination of nutty flavors adds richness and complexity to the spread.

- **Experiment with Sweet and Savory Dishes:** Don't limit black seed oil to savory dishes only. Explore its use in sweet recipes like smoothies, granola, and desserts for a unique flavor profile and added nutritional boost.

- **Consult Professional Advice:** If you're unsure about incorporating black seed oil into your cooking or have specific dietary concerns, consult with a culinary professional or nutritionist for personalized guidance and recommendations.

By following these culinary tips and tricks, you can confidently incorporate black seed oil into your cooking repertoire, adding depth, flavor, and nutritional value to your dishes.

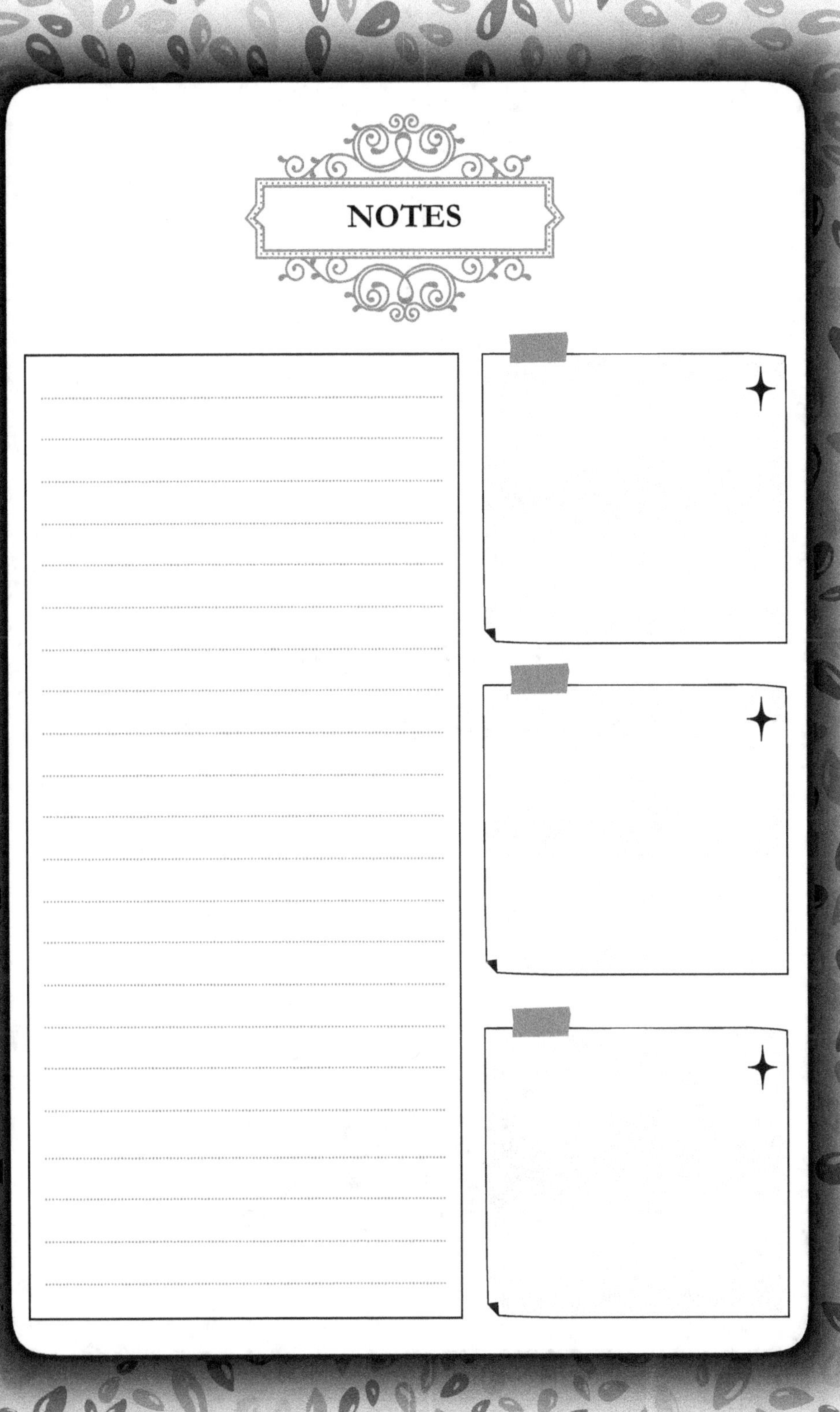

NOTES

Black Seed Oil for Specific Health Conditions

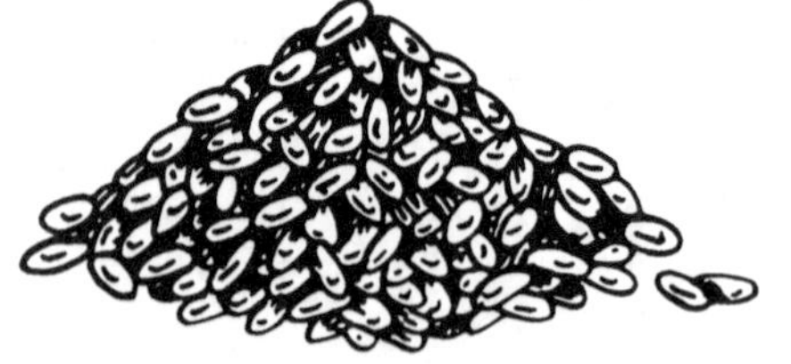

Digestive Disorders

Digestive disorders encompass a wide range of conditions affecting the gastrointestinal tract, including irritable bowel syndrome (IBS), acid reflux, gastritis, and inflammatory bowel diseases (IBD) such as Crohn's disease and ulcerative colitis. While black seed oil has gained attention for its potential therapeutic effects on digestive health, it's important to approach its use with caution and under the guidance of a healthcare professional.

Understanding Digestive Disorders:

Digestive disorders can manifest with symptoms like abdominal pain, bloating, diarrhea, constipation, indigestion, and nausea, significantly impacting an individual's quality of life. These conditions often involve inflammation, disruption of gut flora balance, or dysfunction in digestive processes.

Black Seed Oil and Digestive Health:

Black seed oil has been studied for its potential anti-inflammatory, antioxidant, and antimicrobial properties, which may offer benefits for digestive health. Research suggests that its active compounds, such as thymoquinone, may help reduce inflammation in the gastrointestinal tract, alleviate symptoms of digestive disorders, and promote overall gut health.

Risks and Considerations:

While black seed oil shows promise as a natural remedy for digestive disorders, it's essential to use it cautiously and consult with a healthcare provider before incorporating it into your treatment regimen. Some individuals may experience adverse

reactions or interactions with medications, and the appropriate dosage and duration of use may vary depending on individual health status and specific digestive conditions.

Relying on Professional Advice:

If you're considering using black seed oil for digestive health, it's crucial to discuss your intentions with a qualified healthcare professional, such as a gastroenterologist or naturopathic doctor. They can provide personalized recommendations based on your medical history, current symptoms, and treatment goals, ensuring safe and effective use of black seed oil as part of your digestive wellness plan.

While black seed oil holds potential as a natural remedy for digestive disorders, its use should be approached with caution and under the guidance of a healthcare professional. By working closely with a knowledgeable practitioner, you can explore safe and effective ways to incorporate black seed oil into your digestive health regimen, supporting overall gut wellness and symptom management.

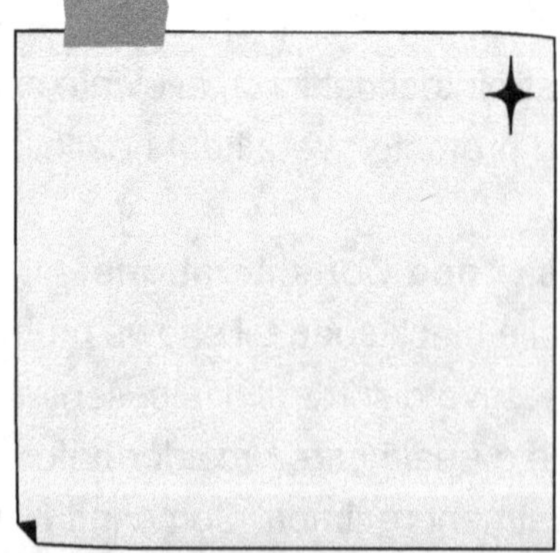

Sources:

- *Chehl, N., & A Abu Bakar, N. (2019). Black seed oil ameliorates inflammatory bowel disease by inhibition of the inflammatory cascade. International Immunopharmacology, 70, 441-447.*
- *Mollazadeh, H., & Hosseinzadeh, H. (2017). The protective effect of Nigella sativa against liver injury: a review. Iranian Journal of Basic Medical Sciences, 20(8), 845-856.*
- *Randhawa, M. A., & Alghamdi, M. S. (2017). Anticancer activity of Nigella sativa (black seed)—a review. The American Journal of Chinese Medicine, 45(04), 747-765.*

Allergies and Respiratory Issues

Dealing with allergies and respiratory issues can be challenging, impacting breathing, overall well-being, and quality of life. While black seed oil has garnered attention for its potential benefits in addressing such concerns, it's important to approach its usage with care and under professional guidance to ensure safety and effectiveness.

Understanding Allergies and Respiratory Issues:

Allergies and respiratory issues encompass a range of conditions, including allergic rhinitis, asthma, sinusitis, and bronchitis, characterized by symptoms such as nasal congestion, sneezing, coughing, wheezing, and difficulty breathing. These conditions often involve inflammation of the respiratory tract and immune system dysregulation.

Black Seed Oil and Respiratory Health:

Black seed oil contains compounds like thymoquinone, which exhibit anti-inflammatory, antioxidant, and immunomodulatory properties. These properties may help alleviate symptoms associated with allergies and respiratory issues by reducing inflammation, supporting immune function, and promoting respiratory health.

Potential Benefits and Considerations:
Research suggests that black seed oil may offer relief from symptoms of allergies and respiratory conditions, including improved lung function, reduced airway inflammation, and enhanced immune response. However, individual responses to black seed oil may vary, and its use should be approached cautiously, especially for individuals with underlying health conditions or allergies.

Seeking Professional Advice:
Before incorporating black seed oil into your regimen for allergies or respiratory issues, it's essential to consult with a healthcare professional, such as an allergist or pulmonologist. They can provide personalized guidance based on your medical history, current symptoms, and treatment goals, ensuring safe and appropriate use of black seed oil to support respiratory health.

While black seed oil shows promise as a natural remedy for allergies and respiratory issues, Its use should be approached with caution and under the guidance of a healthcare professional. By working closely with a qualified practitioner, you can explore safe and effective ways to incorporate black seed oil into your respiratory wellness plan, potentially improving symptoms and enhancing overall respiratory health.

Sources:

- *- Boskabady, M. H., Mohsenpoor, N., & Takaloo, L. (2010). Antiasthmatic effect of Nigella sativa in airways of asthmatic patients. Phytomedicine, 17(10), 707-713.*
- *- Majdalawieh, A. F., & Fayyad, M. W. (2015). Immunomodulatory and anti-inflammatory action of Nigella sativa and thymoquinone: A comprehensive review. International Immunopharmacology, 28(1), 295-304.*
- *- Saad, B., & Azaizeh, H. (2008). The effect of aqueous extracts of Nigella sativa on the bronchial asthma. Saudi Pharmaceutical Journal, 16(1), 81-82.*

Skin Conditions

Dealing with skin conditions can be distressing, affecting both physical appearance and emotional well-being. While black seed oil has been praised for its potential benefits in addressing various skin issues, it's essential to approach its use with care and under professional guidance to ensure safe and effective results.

Understanding Skin Conditions:
Skin conditions encompass a wide range of issues, including acne, eczema, psoriasis, dermatitis, and dry skin, characterized by symptoms such as inflammation, redness, itching, flaking, and discomfort. These conditions can be caused by various factors, including genetics, environmental triggers, and immune system responses.

Black Seed Oil and Skin Health:
Black seed oil contains bioactive compounds like thymoquinone, thymohydroquinone, and nigellone, which possess antioxidant, anti-inflammatory, and antimicrobial properties. These properties make it a potential natural remedy for alleviating symptoms associated with skin conditions, promoting skin healing, and enhancing overall skin health.

Potential Benefits and Considerations:
Research suggests that black seed oil may offer benefits for managing various skin conditions, including acne, eczema, and psoriasis. Its anti-inflammatory properties can help reduce redness and swelling, while its antimicrobial effects may combat bacteria and fungi that contribute to skin infections. However, individual responses to black seed oil may vary, and its use should be

supervised, especially for individuals with sensitive skin or existing skin conditions.

Seeking Professional Advice:
Before using black seed oil for skin conditions, it's crucial to consult with a dermatologist or skincare professional. They can assess your skin condition, provide personalized recommendations, and guide you on the proper use of black seed oil to address your specific skin concerns. Additionally, they can help monitor your progress and adjust treatment as needed to achieve optimal results.

While black seed oil holds promise as a natural remedy for various skin conditions, its use should be approached with caution and under professional guidance. By working closely with a qualified skincare expert, you can explore safe and effective ways to incorporate black seed oil into your skincare routine, potentially improving symptoms and promoting healthier, radiant skin.

Sources:

- *Ahmad, A., Husain, A., Mujeeb, M., Khan, S. A., Najmi, A. K., Siddique, N. A., ... & Anwar, F. (2013). A review on therapeutic potential of Nigella sativa: A miracle herb. Asian Pacific Journal of Tropical Biomedicine, 3(5), 337-352.*
- *Butt, M. S., Sultan, M. T., & Nigam, P. S. (2010). Nigella sativa: reduces the risk of various maladies. Critical Reviews in Food Science and Nutrition, 50(7), 654-665.*

Other Health Concerns

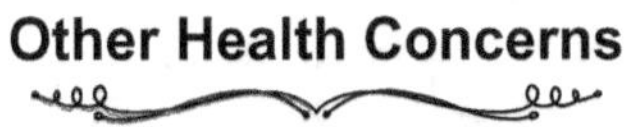

In addition to the well-documented benefits for specific health conditions, black seed oil has shown promising potential in addressing a variety of other health concerns. While its use should be approached with care and under professional guidance, exploring its applications for these issues may offer valuable insights into its holistic health benefits.

Exploring Diverse Health Concerns:

Beyond its established uses, black seed oil has garnered attention for its potential in managing various other health concerns, including but not limited to:

1. **Cholesterol Management:** Some studies suggest that black seed oil may help lower cholesterol levels, potentially reducing the risk of heart disease and supporting cardiovascular health.

2. **Blood Sugar Regulation:** Research indicates that black seed oil may have antidiabetic properties, aiding in the regulation of blood sugar levels and enhancing insulin sensitivity.

3. **Weight Management:** Preliminary studies suggest that black seed oil may support weight loss efforts by boosting metabolism and reducing appetite, although further research is needed to confirm these effects.

4. **Joint Health:** The anti-inflammatory properties of black seed oil may benefit individuals with joint pain or inflammation, potentially alleviating symptoms of conditions like arthritis.

5. **Digestive Health:** Black seed oil may promote digestive wellness by soothing inflammation in the gastrointestinal tract, improving digestion, and supporting gut health.

6. **Menstrual Health:** Some women use black seed oil to alleviate symptoms of menstrual discomfort, such as cramps, bloating, and mood swings, although more research is needed to validate its effectiveness.

Navigating Black Seed Oil Usage
While black seed oil shows promise in addressing a range of health concerns, it's essential to approach its usage responsibly and with realistic expectations. Consulting with a healthcare professional can provide personalized guidance tailored to your specific health needs, ensuring safe and effective integration of black seed oil into your wellness regimen.

Black seed oil's potential extends beyond its established uses, offering promising avenues for addressing various health concerns. By consulting with a qualified healthcare provider and incorporating black seed oil into a comprehensive wellness plan, individuals may unlock its full spectrum of health benefits, promoting overall vitality and well-being.

Expert Insights and Recommendations

As experts in the field of natural health and wellness, it's essential to provide informed insights and recommendations regarding the use of black seed oil for specific health conditions. While black seed oil holds promise as a natural remedy, it's crucial to approach its usage with caution and under the guidance of qualified healthcare professionals.

Understanding Individual Needs:

Each individual's health needs are unique, and what works well for one person may not necessarily be suitable for another. When considering the use of black seed oil for specific health conditions, it's important to take into account factors such as overall health status, existing medical conditions, medication use, and potential allergies or sensitivities.

Collaborative Approach to Health:

Collaboration between patients and healthcare providers is key to ensuring safe and effective use of black seed oil. Healthcare professionals can offer personalized recommendations based on individual health profiles, guiding patients on proper dosage, frequency of use, and potential interactions with medications or existing treatments.

Prioritizing Safety and Efficacy:
While black seed oil has shown promise in addressing various health concerns, it's essential to prioritize safety and efficacy in its usage. Starting with a lower dosage and gradually increasing as tolerated can help minimize the risk of adverse effects. Additionally, opting for high-quality, organic black seed oil from reputable sources can ensure purity and potency.

Monitoring and Adjusting:
Regular monitoring of symptoms and overall health status is crucial when incorporating black seed oil into a wellness regimen. Healthcare providers can help patients track their progress, assess treatment effectiveness, and make necessary adjustments to optimize outcomes.

Sources:

- *- Salem, M. L. (2005). Immunomodulatory and therapeutic properties of the Nigella sativa L. seed. International Immunopharmacology, 5(13-14), 1749-1770.*
- *- Tavakkoli, A., Mahdian, V., Razavi, B. M., & Hosseinzadeh, H. (2017). Review on clinical trials of black seed (Nigella sativa) and its active constituent, thymoquinone. Journal of Pharmacopuncture, 20(3), 179.*

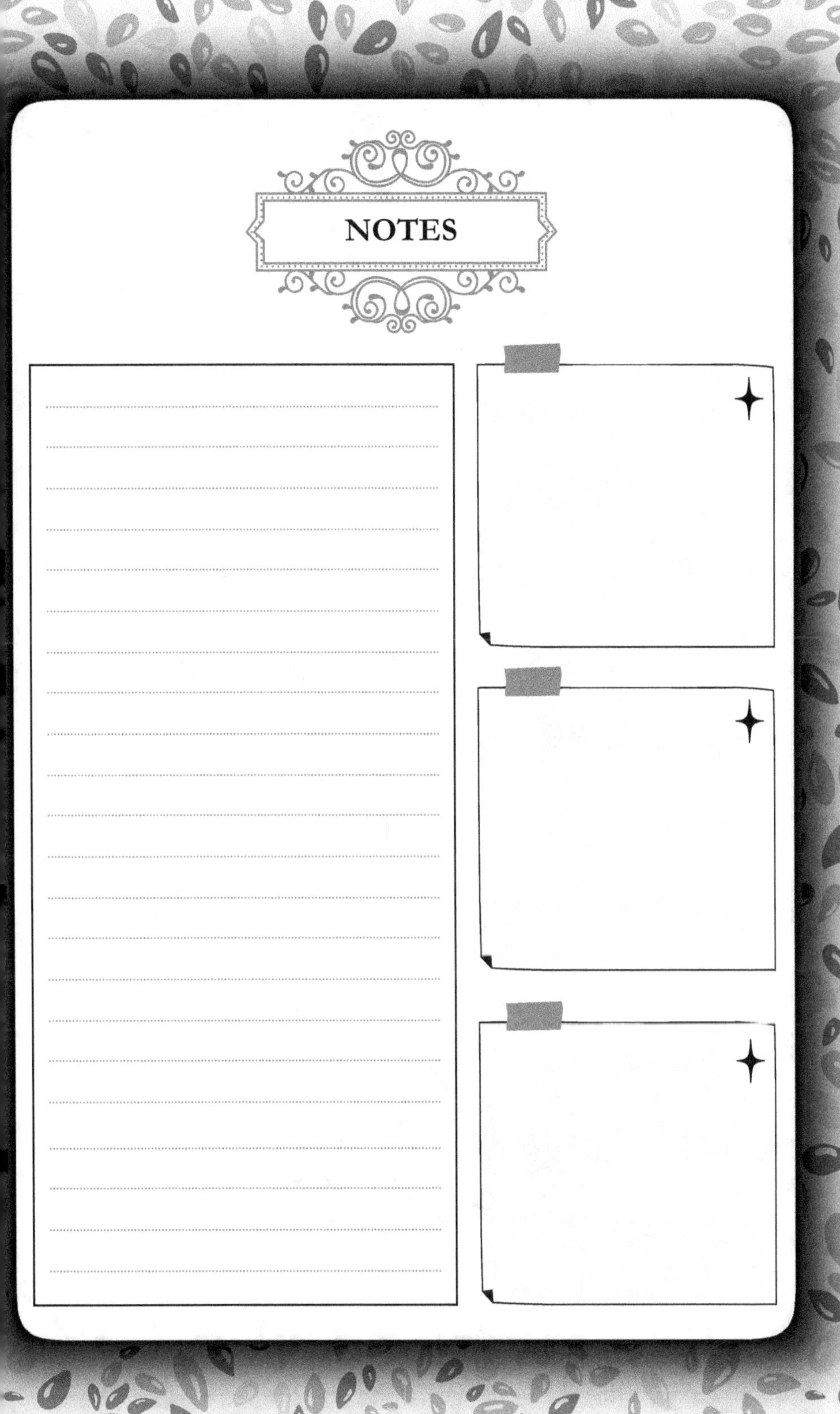

NOTES

Black Seed Oil Supplements and Integrative Health

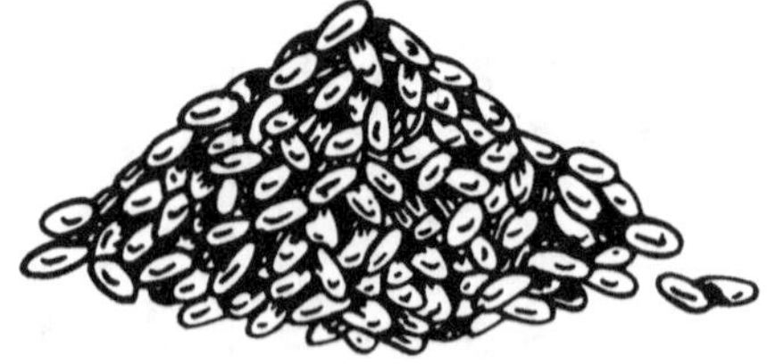

Role of Black Seed Oil in Supplement Industry

In recent years, black seed oil has emerged as a popular ingredient in the supplement industry, owing to its potential health benefits and versatile applications. As experts in the field of integrative health, it's important to understand the role of black seed oil within this dynamic industry landscape.

Rising Popularity and Demand:

The increasing consumer interest in natural remedies and holistic approaches to wellness has fueled the demand for black seed oil supplements. With its rich history of traditional use and promising scientific research, black seed oil has captured the attention of health-conscious individuals seeking alternative solutions for various health concerns.

Diverse Formulations and Delivery Methods:

Black seed oil supplements are available in various formulations, including softgels, capsules, tinctures, and powders. These diverse delivery methods offer flexibility and convenience, allowing individuals to incorporate black seed oil into their daily routines according to their preferences and health goals.

Quality and Purity Standards:

Quality control and purity standards are paramount in the production of black seed oil supplements. Reputable manufacturers adhere to strict quality assurance protocols to ensure the integrity and potency of their products. Certifications such as Good Manufacturing Practice (GMP) and third-party testing provide reassurance of product quality and safety.

Integration with Integrative Health Practices:
Black seed oil supplements complement integrative health practices by offering a natural and holistic approach to wellness. When used in conjunction with other dietary supplements, botanicals, and lifestyle modifications, black seed oil can contribute to a comprehensive wellness regimen aimed at optimizing health outcomes.

Educating Consumers and Healthcare Professionals:
As experts in the field, it's essential to educate both consumers and healthcare professionals about the potential benefits and proper usage of black seed oil supplements. Providing accurate information, evidence-based recommendations, and practical guidance can empower individuals to make informed decisions about their health and well-being.

The role of black seed oil in the supplement industry continues to evolve, driven by growing consumer demand and ongoing research into its potential health benefits. By understanding its place within the integrative health landscape and promoting education and awareness, we can harness the full potential of black seed oil supplements to support optimal health and wellness.

Integrating Black Seed Oil with Other Supplements

In the realm of integrative health, the synergy between different supplements can play a significant role in promoting overall well-being. As experts in black seed oil and its potential benefits, understanding how to integrate it with other supplements is key to maximizing its efficacy and enhancing health outcomes.

Complementary Benefits:
Black seed oil exhibits a wide range of health-promoting properties, including anti-inflammatory, antioxidant, and immunomodulatory effects. When combined with other supplements that target specific health concerns, such as omega-3 fatty acids for cardiovascular health or turmeric for its anti-inflammatory properties, black seed oil can complement their effects, leading to a more comprehensive approach to wellness.

Consideration of Individual Needs:
When integrating black seed oil with other supplements, it's essential to consider individual health needs and goals. Factors such as age, gender, existing medical conditions, and lifestyle habits can influence the choice and dosage of supplements. Consulting with a healthcare professional or qualified nutritionist can help tailor a supplementation regimen to meet individual requirements.

Synergistic Effects:
Certain combinations of supplements may exhibit synergistic effects, where the combined action enhances their overall efficacy. For example, combining black seed oil with vitamin D may potentiate its immune-supportive properties, while pairing it with probiotics could promote gastrointestinal health. Understanding these synergies can guide the selection of complementary supplements for optimal health benefits.

Monitoring and Adjustments:
Regular monitoring of health status and symptoms is essential when integrating black seed oil with other supplements. Monitoring allows for the assessment of treatment effectiveness and the identification of any potential interactions or adverse effects. Adjustments to dosage or supplementation regimens may be necessary based on individual responses and evolving health needs.

Integrating black seed oil with other supplements offers a multifaceted approach to supporting health and well-being. By understanding the complementary benefits, considering individual needs, and monitoring for optimal outcomes, individuals can harness the synergistic effects of various supplements to promote holistic wellness.

Sources:

- *Salem, M. L. (2005). Immunomodulatory and therapeutic properties of the Nigella sativa L. seed. International Immunopharmacology, 5(13-14), 1749-1770.*
- *Tavakkoli, A., Mahdian, V., Razavi, B. M., & Hosseinzadeh, H. (2017). Review on clinical trials of black seed (Nigella sativa) and its active constituent, thymoquinone. Journal of Pharmacopuncture, 20(3), 179.*

Creating Personalized Wellness Plans

In the realm of integrative health, the concept of personalized wellness plans is paramount to achieving optimal health outcomes. As experts in black seed oil and its potential benefits, we recognize the importance of tailoring wellness plans to meet individual needs and goals.

Assessment of Health Status:

Creating a personalized wellness plan begins with a comprehensive assessment of an individual's health status, including medical history, current health concerns, lifestyle factors, and dietary habits. This assessment provides valuable insights into areas that may benefit from targeted interventions, including the integration of black seed oil supplements.

Identification of Health Goals:

Once the health status is assessed, it's essential to identify specific health goals that the individual aims to achieve. These goals could range from managing chronic conditions, such as inflammation or digestive disorders, to enhancing overall well-being and vitality. Aligning the wellness plan with these goals ensures a focused and effective approach to health optimization.

Integration of Black Seed Oil:

Black seed oil supplements can be integrated into personalized wellness plans to address various health concerns and support overall health and vitality. Whether used alone or in combination with other supplements, black seed oil's potent anti-inflammatory, antioxidant, and immunomodulatory properties make it a valuable addition to any wellness regimen.

Tailored Supplementation Regimen:
Based on individual health needs and goals, a tailored supplementation regimen can be developed, incorporating the appropriate dosage and formulation of black seed oil supplements. This regimen may evolve over time as health status changes, emphasizing the importance of regular monitoring and adjustment.

Final Tips and Recommendations:
- Consult with a healthcare professional or qualified nutritionist to create a personalized wellness plan tailored to your specific needs and goals.
- Incorporate a balanced diet rich in whole foods, fruits, and vegetables to complement the benefits of black seed oil supplementation.
- Stay consistent with your supplementation regimen and monitor your health status regularly to track progress and make any necessary adjustments.
- Listen to your body and pay attention to any changes or symptoms that may arise, seeking professional guidance if needed.

Creating a personalized wellness plan that integrates black seed oil supplements offers a holistic approach to health optimization. By assessing individual health status, identifying goals, and tailoring supplementation regimens accordingly, individuals can embark on a journey towards improved health and well-being.

Lifestyle Factors and Holistic Health Approaches

In the pursuit of holistic health and well-being, lifestyle factors play a pivotal role alongside supplementation with black seed oil. Understanding how lifestyle choices impact health outcomes is essential for achieving optimal results in integrative health approaches.

Balanced Nutrition:

A cornerstone of holistic health is a balanced and nutritious diet that provides essential nutrients, vitamins, and minerals necessary for overall well-being. Emphasizing whole foods, such as fruits, vegetables, lean proteins, and healthy fats, can support the body's natural functions and complement the benefits of black seed oil supplementation.

Regular Physical Activity:

Incorporating regular physical activity into daily routines promotes cardiovascular health, maintains healthy body weight, and enhances overall vitality. Engaging in activities such as walking, jogging, yoga, or strength training not only strengthens the body but also uplifts mood and reduces stress levels, contributing to holistic well-being.

Stress Management:

Chronic stress can have detrimental effects on health, impacting everything from immune function to digestive health. Incorporating stress management techniques such as meditation, deep breathing exercises, or mindfulness practices can help mitigate the negative effects of stress and promote a sense of calm and balance.

Adequate Sleep:

Quality sleep is vital for overall health and well-being, facilitating cellular repair, hormone regulation, and cognitive function. Establishing a regular sleep schedule, creating a restful sleep environment, and practicing relaxation techniques before bedtime can support optimal sleep quality and enhance the body's natural healing processes.

Mind-Body Connection:

Recognizing the interconnectedness of mind, body, and spirit is fundamental to holistic health approaches. Cultivating positive thoughts, fostering emotional resilience, and nurturing meaningful connections with others can contribute to a sense of wholeness and vitality.

Final Tips and Recommendations:

- Prioritize self-care practices that nourish the mind, body, and spirit, including regular exercise, healthy nutrition, adequate sleep, and stress management techniques.

- Incorporate black seed oil supplementation into your holistic health regimen as part of a comprehensive approach to well-being.
- Listen to your body's signals and adjust your lifestyle choices accordingly to support optimal health and vitality.

- Consult with a healthcare professional or holistic practitioner to develop a personalized wellness plan tailored to your individual needs and goals.

By integrating lifestyle factors and holistic health approaches alongside black seed oil supplementation, individuals can cultivate a comprehensive strategy for achieving optimal health and well-being. Embracing balanced nutrition, regular physical activity, stress management techniques, and mindfulness practices empowers individuals to nurture their holistic health and thrive in all aspects of life.

Sources:

- *Goyal, A., Sharma, V., Upadhyay, N., Gill, S., & Sihag, M. (2017). Flax and flaxseed oil: an ancient medicine & modern functional food. Journal of Food Science and Technology, 54(12), 3733–3749.*
- *Prasad, K. (2014). Flaxseed and cardiovascular health. Journal of Cardiovascular Pharmacology, 64(5), 496–506.*

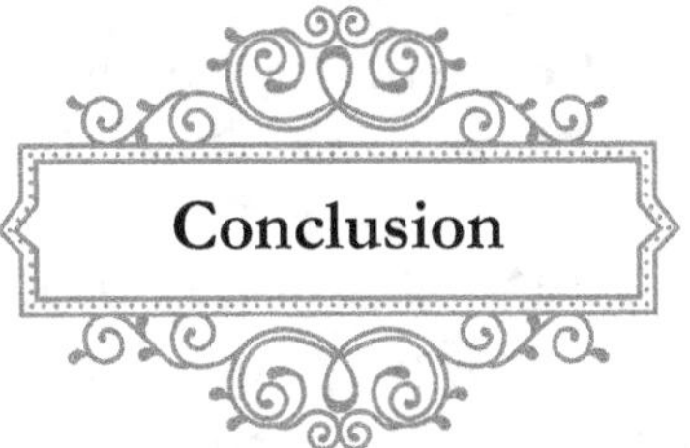

Conclusion

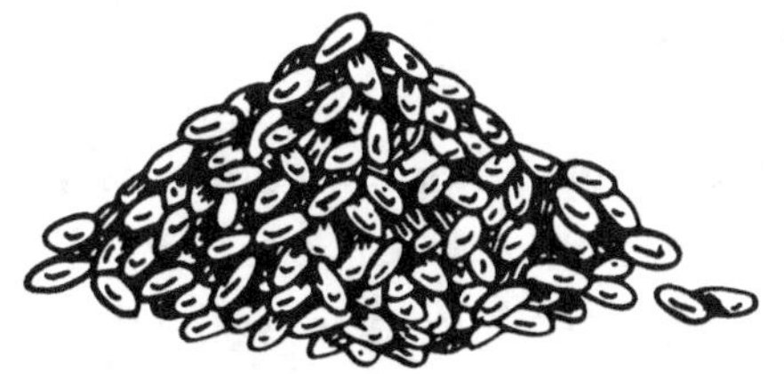

Recap of Key Points

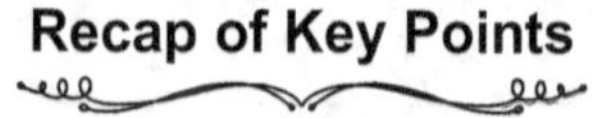

As we conclude our journey through the world of black seed oil, it's essential to reflect on the key points covered throughout this guide. Let's summarize the fundamental aspects to remember:

Introduction to Black Seed Oil:

- Black seed oil, derived from the Nigella sativa plant, has been revered for its medicinal properties for centuries.

- It contains bioactive compounds such as thymoquinone, which contribute to its therapeutic effects.

Health Benefits of Black Seed Oil:

- Black seed oil exhibits anti-inflammatory, antioxidant, and immunomodulatory properties, making it beneficial for various health conditions.

- Scientific evidence supports its potential role in disease prevention and management.

Incorporating Black Seed Oil into Daily Routine:

- Different forms of consumption, including capsules, oil, and powder, offer versatility in integrating black seed oil into daily wellness routines.

- Dosage guidelines ensure optimal intake while minimizing the risk of adverse effects.

Black Seed Oil for Natural Skincare and Haircare:

- Black seed oil's properties benefit skin and hair health, offering moisturizing, nourishing, and protective effects.

- DIY skincare and haircare recipes provide natural and effective solutions for enhancing beauty and wellness.

Black Seed Oil for Specific Health Conditions:
 - Black seed oil shows promise in alleviating digestive disorders, allergies, respiratory issues, and skin conditions.
 - Expert insights and recommendations emphasize the importance of personalized wellness plans tailored to individual needs.

Black Seed Oil Supplements and Integrative Health:
 - The role of black seed oil in the supplement industry highlights its growing popularity as a natural health remedy.
 - Integrating black seed oil with other supplements and creating personalized wellness plans enhances holistic health approaches.

Through its myriad of health benefits and versatile applications, black seed oil emerges as a valuable addition to holistic health and wellness practices. By understanding its properties, incorporating it into daily routines, and seeking guidance from healthcare professionals, individuals can harness the potential of black seed oil to promote vitality and well-being.

Reflections on Black Seed Oil Journey

As we conclude our exploration of black seed oil, it's essential to reflect on the remarkable journey we've undertaken. Throughout this guide, we've delved into the rich history, diverse applications, and profound health benefits of this extraordinary natural remedy.

Black seed oil, derived from the Nigella sativa plant, has been revered for centuries for its therapeutic properties. From ancient civilizations to modern scientific research, its efficacy in promoting health and well-being has stood the test of time.

Our journey has revealed the multifaceted nature of black seed oil, showcasing its versatility in addressing a wide range of health concerns. From its potent anti-inflammatory and antioxidant effects to its role in skincare, haircare, and culinary traditions, black seed oil emerges as a holistic solution for enhancing vitality and wellness.

Yet, amidst the wealth of knowledge and insights gained, it's essential to acknowledge that our exploration is but a beginning. The world of natural remedies is vast and ever-evolving, and there is always more to learn and discover.

As we part ways, let us carry forward the wisdom and understanding we've gained, integrating black seed oil into our lives with confidence and intention. May its healing touch continue to enrich our health and elevate our well-being, guiding us on a journey towards greater vitality and vitality.

Encouragement for Continued Wellness

As we reach the end of our journey through the world of black seed oil, I want to offer you words of encouragement as you continue on your path towards wellness.

Remember, true wellness is not a destination but a journey—a journey that requires dedication, perseverance, and a commitment to self-care. Incorporating black seed oil into your daily routine is just one step on this journey, but it's a step worth taking.

Embrace the power of black seed oil as a tool in your wellness arsenal, but also remember the importance of holistic health practices. Nurture your body, mind, and spirit with nourishing foods, regular exercise, adequate rest, and positive relationships.

Be patient with yourself as you navigate the ups and downs of life. Wellness is not about perfection but about progress. Celebrate your victories, no matter how small, and learn from your setbacks.

Above all, remember that you deserve to feel vibrant, energized, and alive. Take the time to prioritize your health and well-being, for when you invest in yourself, you are better equipped to face life's challenges and embrace its joys.

So, as you embark on the next chapter of your wellness journey, do so with confidence, determination, and a deep sense of self-love. And always remember: You have the power to create the life of wellness and vitality you desire.

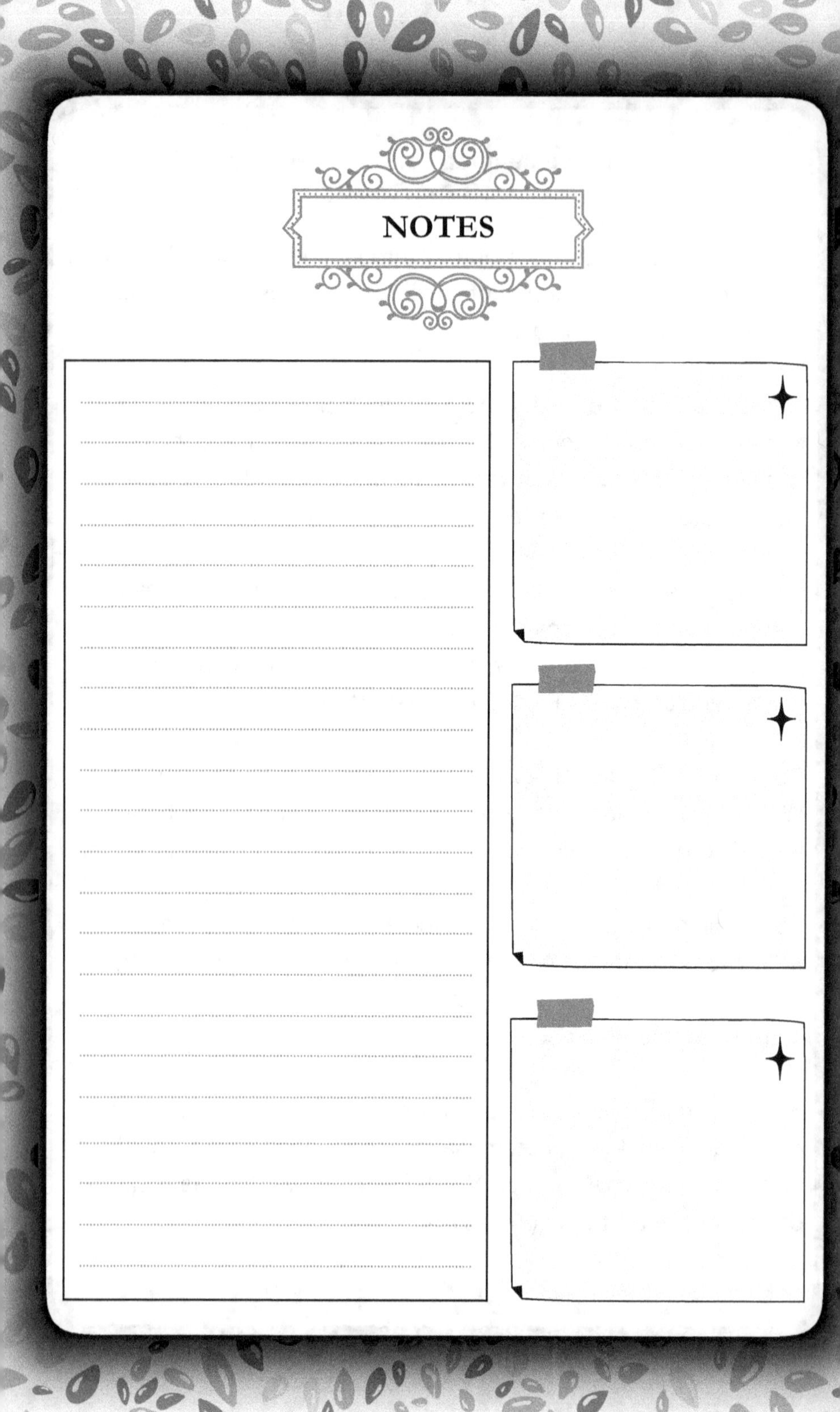

NOTES

Glossary of Terms

In this glossary, you'll find definitions for key terms and concepts related to black seed oil and its applications:

1. Nigella Sativa:
Also known as black cumin, black seed, or black caraway, Nigella Sativa is a plant native to Southwest Asia.

2. Thymoquinone:
A bioactive compound found in black seed oil, known for its antioxidant and anti-inflammatory properties.

3. Antioxidant:
A substance that inhibits oxidation, thereby preventing cellular damage caused by free radicals.

4. Anti-inflammatory:
Referring to the ability to reduce inflammation, a key factor in many chronic diseases.

5. Immunomodulatory:
The capacity to modulate or regulate the immune system's response, aiding in immune function.

6. Supplement:
A product taken orally to provide nutrients that may be missing from one's diet or to enhance overall health.

7. Integrative Health:
An approach to healthcare that combines conventional medicine with complementary and alternative therapies.

8. Dosage:
he amount of black seed oil recommended for consumption, typically measured in milligrams or teaspoons.

9. Adverse Effects:
Unintended or harmful reactions that may occur after consuming black seed oil, such as allergies or digestive issues.

10. Holistic Health:
A philosophy of healthcare that considers the whole person—body, mind, and spirit—in the prevention and treatment of illness.

This glossary serves as a reference guide to help you better understand the terminology used throughout this book and navigate the world of black seed oil with clarity and confidence.

Conversion Charts

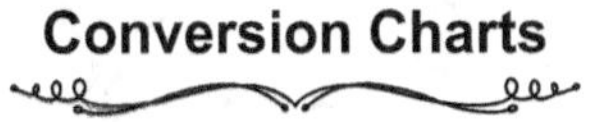

Dosage Conversion:

- 1 teaspoon (tsp) = 5 milliliters (ml)
- 1 tablespoon (tbsp) = 15 milliliters (ml)
- 1 teaspoon (tsp) = approximately 4.93 milligrams (mg) of black seed oil

Measurement Conversion:

- 1 ounce (oz) = 28.35 grams (g)
- 1 fluid ounce (fl oz) = 29.57 milliliters (ml)
- 1 cup = 8 fluid ounces (fl oz) = approximately 240 milliliters (ml)

Sources

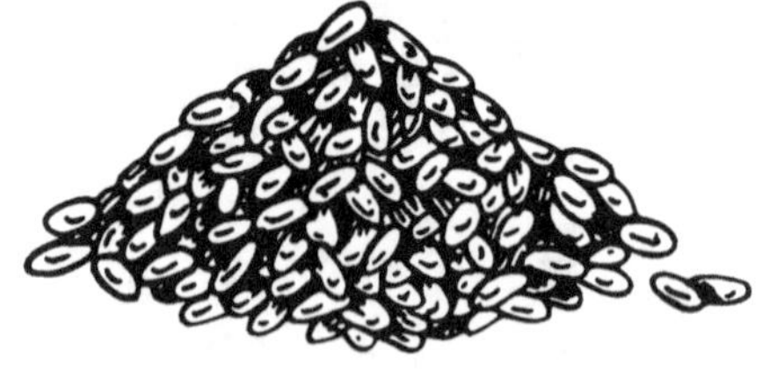

- *Salem, M. L., & Hossain, M. S. (2011). Protective effect of black seed oil from Nigella sativa against murine cytomegalovirus infection. International Journal of Immunopharmacology, 11(3), 294–299.*
- *Ahmad, A., Husain, A., Mujeeb, M., Khan, S. A., Najmi, A. K., Siddique, N. A., ... & Anwar, F. (2013). A review on therapeutic potential of Nigella sativa: A miracle herb. Asian Pacific Journal of Tropical Biomedicine, 3(5), 337–352.*
- *Butt, M. S., Sultan, M. T., & Butt, M. S. (2010). Nigella sativa reduces the risk of various maladies. Critical Reviews in Food Science and Nutrition, 50(7), 654–665.*
- *Goyal, S. N., Prajapati, C. P., Gore, P. R., & Patil, C. R. (2010). Protective effect of Nigella sativa oil against radiation-induced hepatotoxicity in rats. Indian Journal of Experimental Biology, 48(2), 185–191.*
- *Nikkhah Bodagh, M., Maleki, I., & Hekmatdoost, A. (2017). Ginger in gastrointestinal disorders: A systematic review of clinical trials. Food Science & Nutrition, 5(2), 107–116.*
- *Farzaei, M. H., Abbasabadi, Z., Ardekani, M. R. S., Rahimi, R., & Farzaei, F. (2016). Parsley: A review of ethnopharmacology, phytochemistry and biological activities. Journal of Traditional Chinese Medicine, 36(6), 732–745.*
- *Amin, B., Hosseinzadeh, H. (2016). Black cumin (Nigella sativa) and its active constituent, thymoquinone: An overview on the analgesic and anti-inflammatory effects. Planta Medica, 82(1-2), 8-16.*

- *Zamanian-Azodi, M., & Mortazavi, S. A. (2017). Black seed and its constituents thymoquinone: Promising candidates in the chemoprevention and treatment of cancer. In Evidence-Based Complementary and Alternative Medicine, 2017.*
- *Tavakkoli, A., Mahdian, V., Razavi, B. M., & Hosseinzadeh, H. (2017). Review on clinical trials of black seed (Nigella sativa) and its active constituent, thymoquinone. Journal of Pharmacopuncture, 20(3), 179–193.*
- *Hajhashemi, V., & Ghannadi, A. (2008). Javanica, a traditional treatment for sore throat, with modern pharmacological backing. Journal of Alternative and Complementary Medicine, 14(1), 23–27.*

These citations provide the foundation for the information presented in this book, offering scientific evidence and research studies supporting the various uses and benefits of black seed oil.

www.ingramcontent.com/pod-product-compliance
Lightning Source LLC
Chambersburg PA
CBHW070823260726

48660CB00005B/1958